FOOD

Hacks, Helps & Hints

Compiled by

C.A. Simonson

Printed in the United States of America.

ISBN: 9781731336347

This book is composed of tips, hints, hacks, and helps to make preparing food easier, quicker, and more flavorful. These tips were gathered from all over the nation. They have been gleaned from my own experiments which have survived, from relatives, old church cookbooks, multiple websites, and from wonderful cooks and chefs who have tried and found success.

No claims are intended to the effectiveness of any suggestions.

Table of Contents

The first part of the twentieth century in 1900s, what we now think of as "hacks" were called "kinks." Some of the ideas in this book came from *Household Discoveries and Mrs. Curtis's Cookbook* in 1908 with ideas supplied from over 25,000 practical homemakers.

✠

A hack refers to any trick, shortcut, skill, or novelty method that increases productivity and efficiency.

✠

In our busy daily living, we all need shortcuts to make our time more efficient and productive. If a simple tip helps make our food quicker, so much the better. An added pleasure is to find it tastier and maybe even healthier.

I hope you find some tips useful, and maybe get a chuckle from a few *Did You Know* trivia facts.

C.A. Simonson

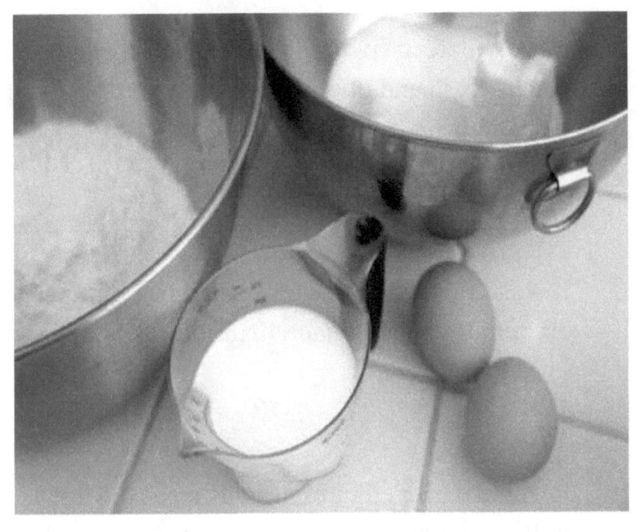

Eggs & Dairy

DID YOU KNOW?

Milk will keep five days past its sell-by date. If it smells fresh and doesn't look separated, it's still okay to drink.

✠

It was said that Cleopatra soaked in a milk bath 30 minutes a day to gain luxurious, soft skin.

✠

In some world cultures such as areas of China, milk is viewed as a form of excrement and abhor drinking it.

✠

Butter was used as food by ancient tribes of Asiatic India, as well as for burning in primitive lamps and smeared on the skin to protect from the cold.

EGGS & DAIRY

1. How old is the egg? Place it in a bowl of cold water. If it lays on its side, it's fresh. If it stands at an angle, it is around three days old; if it stands on end, it is about ten days old.

2. Eggs will last three weeks PAST the sell-by date. (A protective coating during processing prevents bacteria).

3. Make a sunny-side-up egg by frying until the white cooks, and then covering the pan with a lid and removing from heat. The steam cooks the egg yolk without flipping.

4. Poke a hole in the egg yolk if microwaving to keep it from exploding.

5.   Poach an egg in the microwave by placing it in a bowl with a pad of butter. Cover it slightly with water. Cover the bowl and microwave 60-90 seconds.

6.   Make a perfect poached egg by adding a teaspoon of white vinegar to the simmering water. It keeps the yolk from shredding.

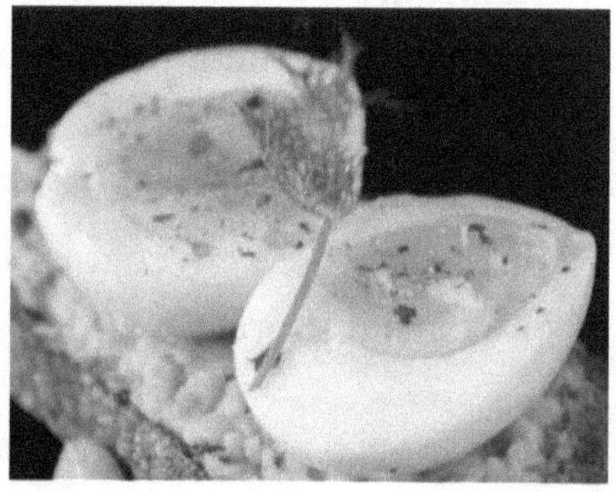

7.   For the perfect hard-boiled egg, bring the water to a boil, then turn off the heat. Let the eggs sit in the water for twelve minutes, and then rinse in cold water.

8.   Keep hardboiled egg yolks from crumbling by dipping the knife in water before slicing.

9. Keep the crust of your quiche crisp by sprinkling Parmesan cheese on the bottom crust before pouring in the egg mixture.

10. Separate eggs easily by putting the raw egg in a plastic baggie. Cut off a corner and let the white seep through.

11. Add a little milk or cream to scrambled eggs for fluffier eggs and omelets.

12. Another way to get fluffy scrambled eggs-- Add WATER to eggs and whip with a fork. Cook in bacon grease and stir constantly.-Jan Gallagher/MO

13. To get cold eggs to room temperature, put them in a bowl of warm water for 10-15 minutes.

14. A little vinegar added to the water while boiling hard-boiled eggs will prevent the eggs from cracking.

15. Put a thumbtack in an egg before boiling to keep it from cracking.

16. Put cooked egg yolks in a zip-lock baggy. Seal and mash. Add mayonnaise and other ingredients for deviled eggs. Keep mashing to mix together. Cut off a corner of the baggy and squeeze the mixture onto halved hard-boiled eggs. Makes for easy preparation and cleanup.

17. Add a drop of food coloring into the boiling water when hard-boiling eggs as a reminder of which are cooked or raw.

18. Keep cream sauce from curdling by using real heavy cream (not milk).

19. When eggs are on sale, buy them up. Crack each egg into an ice cube tray, and then freeze for later use.

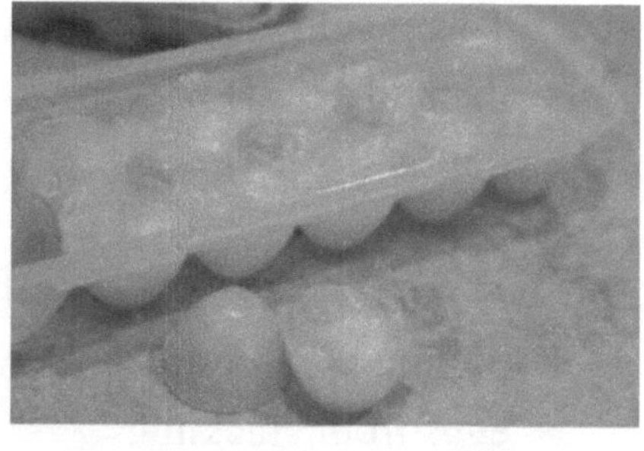

20. When a recipe calls for real butter, use real butter. Substituting margarine or shortening will change the texture, taste, and consistency of the recipe.

21. Butter can be frozen. Unsalted butter keeps longer frozen then salted butter.

22. Soften hard butter by covering it with a warm glass.

23. To get a stick of butter at room temperature, put in the microwave for 10-12 seconds.

24. To prevent butter from scorching or over-browning in the pan, add a drop of lemon juice.

25. You may like fruit on your cereal. Make it even healthier and tastier by drizzling with

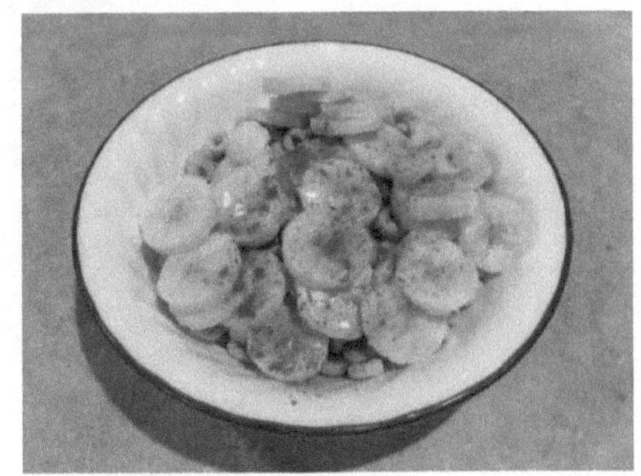

honey (instead of sugar) and sprinkle cinnamon over it!

26. Spray your cheese grater with oil for easier cheese grating.

27. Cold cheese grates easier than warm cheese.

28. Cheese is aged; if dry or moldy spots show up, simply cut them off. It is still good to eat.

29. Store opened chunks of cheese in aluminum foil. It will stay fresher much longer and not mold.

30. Cheese can be frozen but will dry out quickly once thawed.

15

Fruit & Nuts

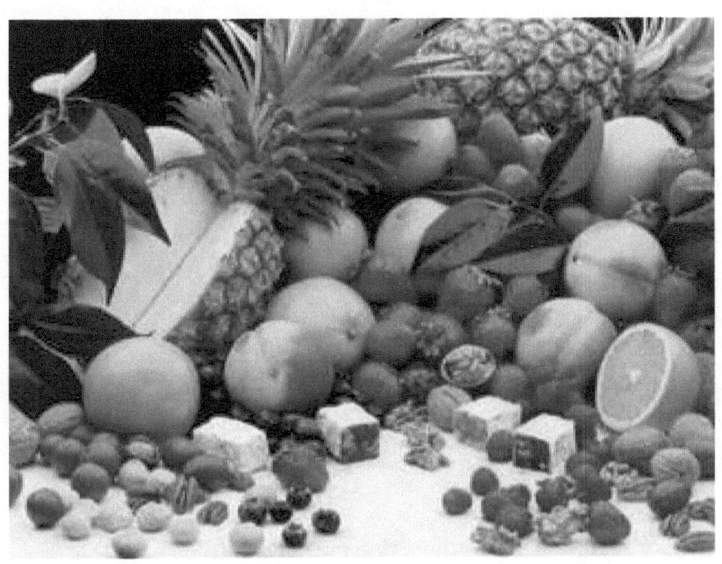

DID YOU KNOW?

Bananas are considered the world's most popular fruit. Its 'tree' is actually the world's largest "herb." There are more than 1000 species of bananas.

✠

A pineapple is actually a bunch of berries that grow together. They got their name from their resemblance to pine cones. Pineapples are considered a symbol of hospitality.

✠

The top three healthiest fruits are the grapefruit followed by the pineapple, and then the avocado. *(healthline.com)

✠

A fruit is the seed-bearing portion of a plant, while a vegetable is the remainder, like a root, leaf, or stem. A berry is a "fleshy fruit that has multiple seeds on the inside." Hmmm…that means squash, cucumbers, and peppers are fruit, while melon and bananas are berries? What are strawberries then? Just a growth of the stem.

FRUIT & NUTS

How to Pick Good Ones

31. For a good cantaloupe, look for close netting pattern. The spaces between the netting should be yellow or yellow-green and a flat spot (where it sat on the ground). Smell it. It should have a very fruity odor.

32. A ripe watermelon has some yellow coloring on one side. If it's white or light green, it is not ripe.

33. Look for avocados with the pebbly skin appearance instead of a smooth skin. They will richer and more buttery tasting.

34. Look for berries that have deep color, not too firm, but not too soft.

35. Get more juice from any citrus fruit by microwaving for 20-30 seconds, then roll it on the counter.

36. Lemon or lime juice squeezed over fruit will keep their color.

37. Bananas left in a bunch ripen quickly. Separate in order to keep them longer.

38. A pinch of salt added to very sour fruits while cooking will reduce the amount of sugar needed to sweeten them.

39. A straw will hull strawberries with ease. Poke the straw through the bottom of the berry up through the leaves.

40. Remove the pit of an avocado by cutting the avocado in half and sticking a knife in the pit.

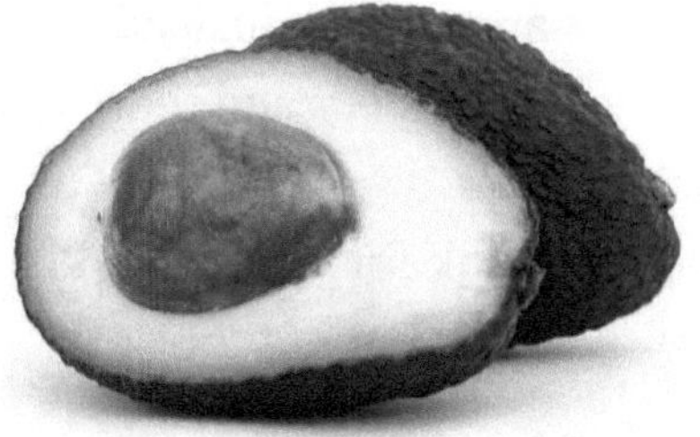

41. Score the avocado into cubes while in the peel and then remove easily with a spoon.

42. Keep an avocado fresh longer by keeping the pit intact when storing it.

43. An ordinary paper clip will easily pit cherries.

44. Bananas can be frozen, although they will turn brown/black. They are still great for smoothies or baking and the flavor has not been lost. It's even better.

Picture by C.A. Simonson

45. Use a spoon to peel the fuzzy skin from a kiwi fruit.

46. Keep fresh berries from the store to last longer by washing them in hot water, and then store in the refrigerator.

47. Sweeten out-of-season fruit by adding 2 Tablespoons of dry lemonade along with sugar.

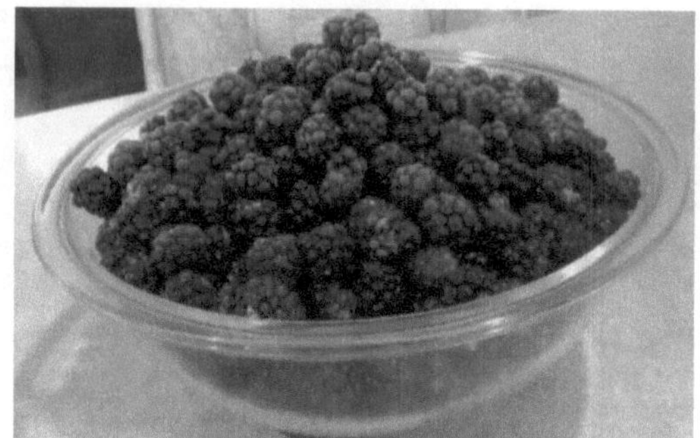

Picture by C.A. Simonson

48.   Nuts keep fresh best in the freezer.

49.   Enhance the flavor of nuts by toasting lightly before using in recipes. Put them on a baking sheet and bake at 300 degrees for about 5-8 minutes.

50.   Make a vinaigrette by using orange or pineapple juice. Add a little olive oil, 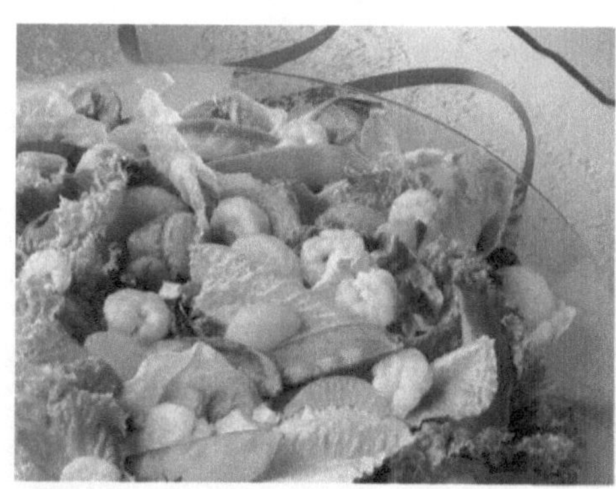 nutmeg, and honey for a fresh taste.

51. Liven up a fruit salad with grated ginger, chopped fresh mint, or toasted coconut.

52. For a simple holiday salad, chop 1 bag of fresh cranberries, 1-2 oranges, and 1-2 apples in a food processor. Add 1 sugar to taste. Store in refrigerator. (Optional: Add miniature marshmallows and chopped walnuts). This is a favorite in our household on Thanksgiving – handed down from my mother's side.

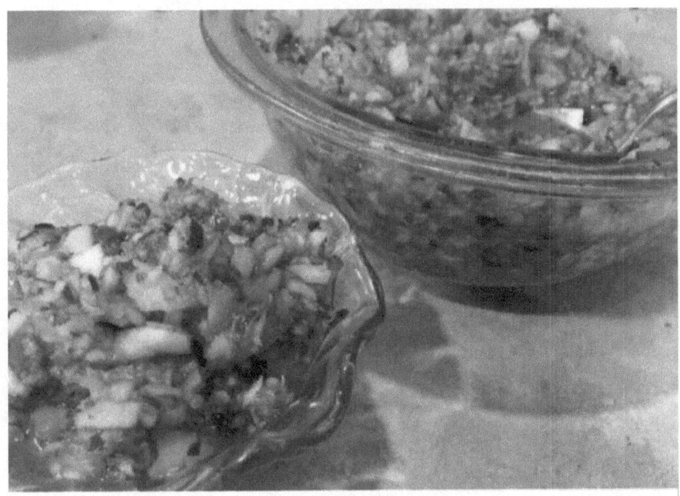

Picture by C.A. Simonson

FOOD HORROR STORIES

A story my late Aunt Verna told about the demise of her lemon pie:

"The Sunshine Club met once a month. We took turns bringing dessert. I slaved all morning to make a good lemon pie for the group. When it was finished, I took a mat and set it on top of the car to cool.

Since our car was headed the wrong way, hubby thought he would be nice and turn the car around, so I could drive straight out. He didn't realize my pie was sitting on top. Well, guess where my pie went...right in the dirt!

One of my cousins said she remembered her dad always liked to eat a slice of cheese with his apple pie. She had the bright idea of putting the cheese slices on top of the apples and baking it in with the pie. Her dad said, "I'll take mine on the side from now on. "

When I was 8-years-old, I decided to make my father his favorite sandwich – Braunschweiger and cheese. My favorite was peanut butter and jelly. Why not put it all together? He ate the sandwich and gracefully with a grimace, told me it was the best one he'd ever eaten.

Vegetables & Pasta

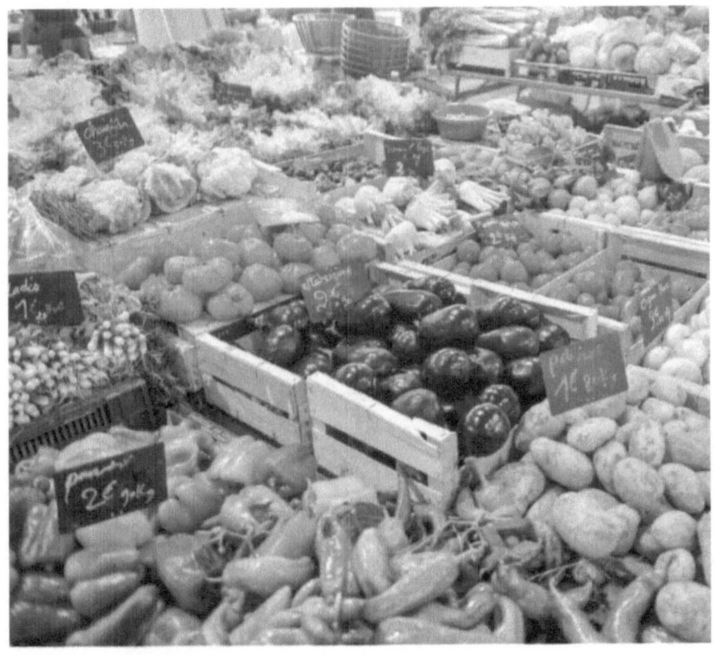

DID YOU KNOW?

Scientists discovered that running electricity through mushrooms can more than double their production, a fact that had been known to Japanese farmers for generations.

✠

There are more than 200 varieties of potatoes sold in the United States.

✠

In preparing French fries at a New York restaurant in 1853, American chef George Crum could not please the customer. The guest complained they were not crispy enough – so Crum sought sliced them ridiculously thin and deep-fried them. Voila! Potato chips – by accident and revenge.

✠

Henry J. Heinz began making ketchup in 1876 but he was neither the inventor nor the first to bottle it. His recipe remains the same to this day.

Tomatoes were once thought to be poisonous because they belong to the nightshade family of plants.

VEGETABLES & PASTA

How to Pick Good Ones

53.   White Russet potatoes are best for baking, but also make fluffy white mashed potatoes; red potatoes are better for salads, soups and escalloped potatoes. Yukon Golds are all-purpose and can be used for anything.

54.   Bi-color corn is the sweetest. Look for smaller kernels for real tender corn. Large kernel corn can become milky, hard and tough.

55.   For great tender asparagus, select young, smaller stalks. Break the fresh spear at the top where it's tender. At the point it won't break easily is where it becomes woody at the bottom.

56. Look for pea pods that are not swollen with peas. Younger peas are more tender and sweeter.

57. When selecting sweet onions, look for flatter onions. They are sweeter than rounded onions with peaks.

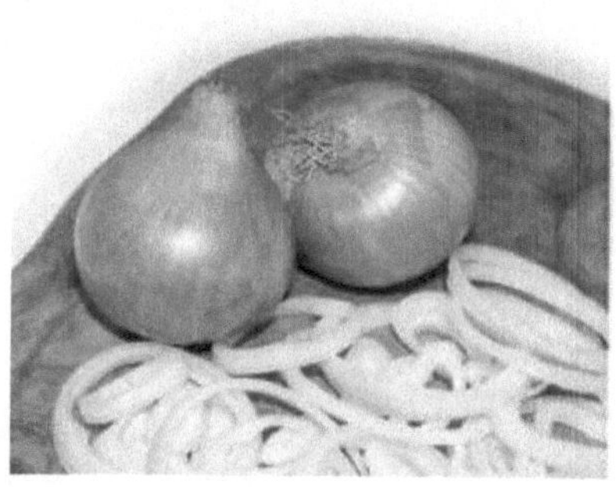

58. Vidalia and Walla Walla onions are the sweetest and mildest – best for salads or onion rings. White or yellow onions are more pungent and keep that flavor while cooking. Red onions can have a peppery taste. White onions are strong but can be used for potato salad or put on hotdogs.

59. If you can smell strong onion odor in the store, it's likely that the onions are close to spoiling. Choose one with tight outer layers.

60.   Choose a good head of lettuce by feeling for the heaviest one.

61.   Beefsteak tomatoes have a mild taste and are best for salsas and hamburger toppings. Meaty Roma tomatoes (shown) are best for making into sauce, having a tangier flavor.

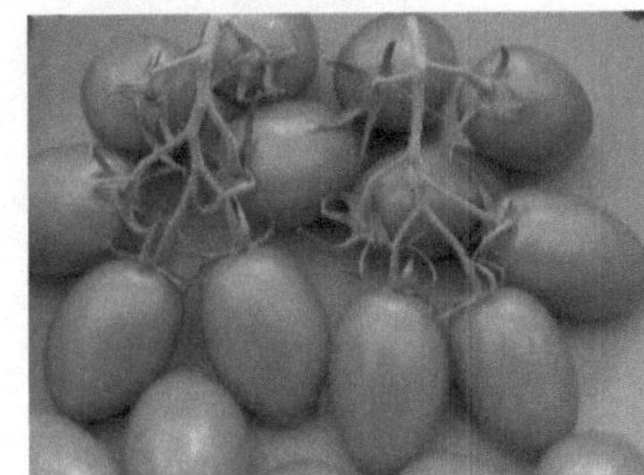

62.   Toss raw veggies in olive oil before seasoning with salt and pepper, and then roast. They're more evenly seasoned.

63.   Drizzle butter or oil over boiled vegetables to keep them moist and flavorful.

64.   Cook vegetables that grow above ground without a lid; vegetables that grow underground, cover the pot.

65.   "Salt in the water can toughen vegetables when cooking. Add it toward the end for more tenderness.

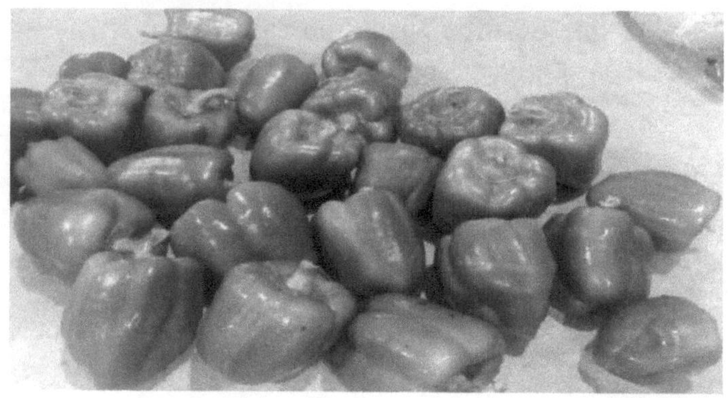

Picture by C.A. Simonson

66.   Peppers with four bumps on the bottom are sweeter and better for eating fresh. Peppers with three bumps are firmer, and better for cooking and making stuffed peppers (however, the four bumps stand up better).

67.   If more oil is needed when sautéing vegetables, add vegetable stock instead of oil. It cuts down on calories, but provides moisture needed.

68.   Potatoes soaked in salt water for twenty
      minutes before baking will bake more
      rapidly.

69.   Cook potatoes and other root vegetables
      faster: cut them up into smaller pieces and
      then let them stand in hot water a few
      minutes after peeling.

70.   A few drops of lemon juice or vinegar
      added to boiled potatoes when draining
      will make them extra white when mashed.

71.   Sprouted
      potatoes
      with eyes
      are still
      good to eat
      if the
      sprouts
      aren't too
      large. If
      the potato has soft spots, however, it is
      ready for planting.

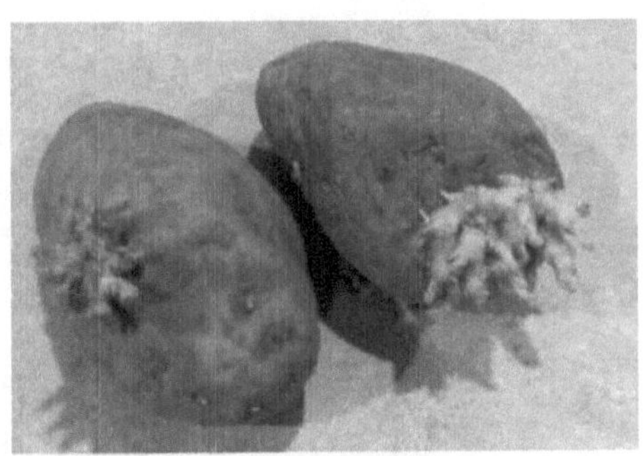

Picture by C.A. Simonson

72.   Mashed potatoes done before the meat?
      Keep them hot by placing a dishtowel over
      the pot, and then cover with the lid. It
      keeps them fluffy and hot.

73.   For creamier, more buttery mashed
      potatoes, melt the butter and add it before
      adding the milk when whipping.

74.   Make French fries taste crisp like
      restaurant-made. Soak the potato strips in
      salty water for an hour before deep-frying.
      Pat dry, and then put into a deep fryer.

75.   Crisp celery stalks by placing
      them upright in a container of
      cold, salty water in the
      refrigerator.

76.   Microwaving a cob of corn in its
      husk will allow it to slip right out. (Make
      sure you have on oven gloves)!

77.   Chili peppers too spicy? Remove seeds
      before using.

78.   Onions do not have to be refrigerated until sliced. Keep them in a dry, dark place. Light makes them bitter.

79.   Onions and potatoes both release moisture and gases that will cause each other to spoil fast. Store them separately to keep them longer.

80.   If a recipe calls for an onion, but doesn't specify, yellow onions are your best choice. They are the standard cooking onion.

81.   If the onion is too strong, tame its pungency by soaking in a container of cold water, and then slice very thin.

82.   Caramelize onions quickly to a golden brown by adding a little baking soda when frying in butter.

83.   Cutting off the root of the onion before slicing will prevent tears.

84.   Make a wonderfully succulent roasted onion. Pull off the outer skin, and then put a pat of butter between each layer. Wrap the whole onion in foil and roast on the grill or in a hot oven.-David Clausen/ OR

85.   Make more "pickles" by adding fresh cucumbers to the brine of an almost-empty pickle jar. (Try other veggies too).

86.   Slice cucumbers thin and add apple cider vinegar, sugar, salt and pepper to taste for sleepy appetites.

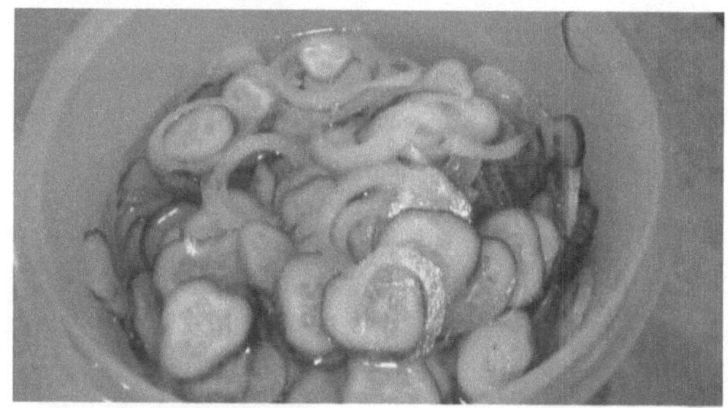

Picture by C.A. Simonson

87.   Rice vinegar gives a more delicate flavor to cucumbers than apple cider vinegar.

Barbara Clausen, CA

88. If you like fried zucchini or green tomatoes, try frying sliced cucumbers. Coat in flour; fry in butter.

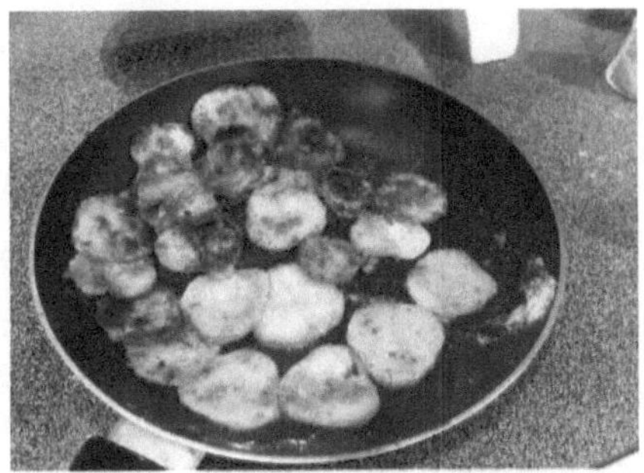

Picture by C.A. Simonson

89. Put one teaspoon of sugar in the water when boiling corn cobs (not salt) for wonderful tasting sweet corn. (Salt toughens kernels).

90. Use your muffin tin to balance stuffed peppers.

91. Remove the core of lettuce by slamming the core end hard on the counter. It will pop right out.

92. For crispier lettuce, remove the core, rinse in cold water, shake it well, and then store in a covered container in the refrigerator.

93. Lettuce that has brown leaves on the outside is still good on the inside. Strip away the wilted leaves, rinse in cold water, drain well, and store in a tight container.

94. Add salt to salad greens to prevent wilting.

95. Eggplant can have bitter juices. Sprinkle salt on the slices and stand vertically in a rack placed in a shallow pan. Let sit ½ hour before cooking to get rid of the bitterness.

96. Keep cauliflower white by adding milk to the water in which it is boiled.

97. Mashed cauliflower tastes and looks like mashed potatoes.

98. Add 1 tsp. of baking soda to cauliflower when cooking or steaming keeps its white color and reduces its odor.

99. Double the life of vine-ripened tomatoes by storing on the counter upside down.

100. Set bananas beside green tomatoes on the counter to help them ripen quickly.

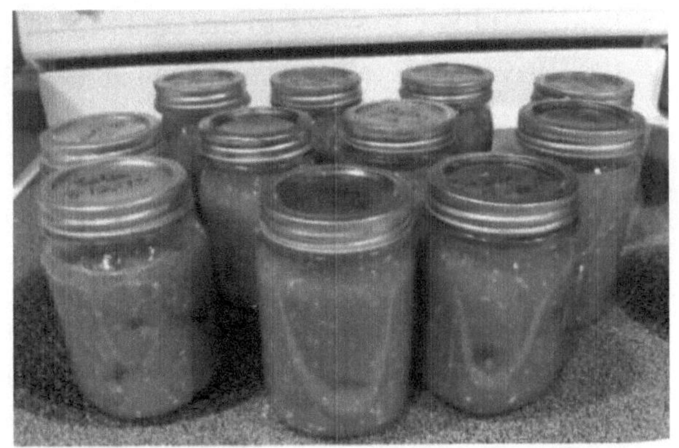

Picture by C.A. Simonson

101. How long can home-canned tomatoes last? I've kept some for up to three years. If the seal is intact, and pops when opened, contents should be good. If the lid doesn't pop, or juice foams, bubbles, or smells bad – throw it away.

102. Peel tomatoes easily by blanching – put them in a pot of semi-boiling water for 15-30 seconds, then slip into an ice-cold bath. Skins slip right off.

103. Add 1-2 Tbsp. of margarine or butter each half of a scooped-out spaghetti squash. Sprinkle liberally with garlic salt and then bake. Add ½ cup water to the baking pan, then cover with foil to steam the squash all around.

104. Don't bother to shell fresh peas. After sorting out bad ones, throw them into boiling water. When they are done, the pods will rise to the surfaces leaving all the peas at the bottom. They'll keep better flavor too.

105. Beets and hummus make a great veggie dip. Terri Lee/CO

106. Cook pasta for salads al dente (slightly chewy). This allows the pasta to absorb some of the dressing and not become mushy.

107. Do not rinse button mushrooms – it makes them mushy. Remove dirt by dabbing with a dry cloth or peeling the outer layer.

108. Rinse wild morel mushrooms in salty water, and then store in paper towels and store in the refrigerator until used.

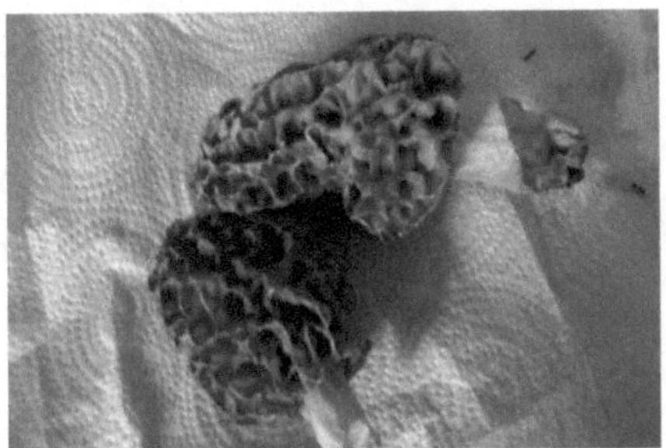

Picture by C.A. Simonson

109. Keep cold appetizers cool by placing the bowl on a bed of ice.

110. When cooking cabbage, place a small cup half full of vinegar on the stove near the cabbage to absorb the odor.

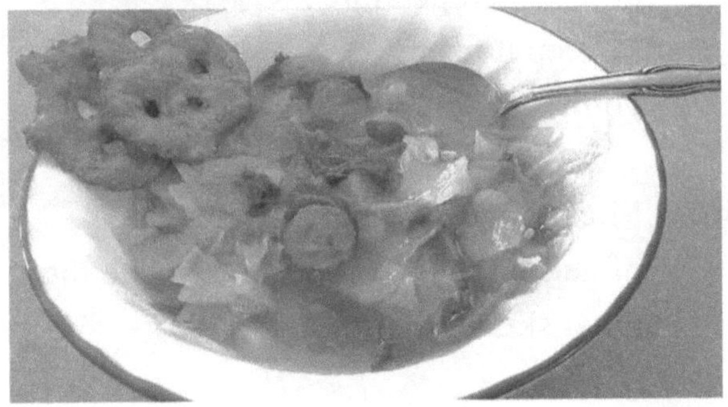

Picture by C.A. Simonson

111. Add 1 tsp. baking soda to cabbage when cooking to tenderize the leaves.

112. Paprika added to any breading mixture will give it a golden-brown color and add potassium to your diet.

113. Keep fresh herbs all winter by chopping and placing in ice cube trays with olive oil. Freeze until needed.

114. Store fresh herbs in a glass partially filled with water – just as you would flowers. If put in the refrigerator, make sure it's away from walls that freeze.

115. Always store garlic at room temperature to keep it from going rancid.

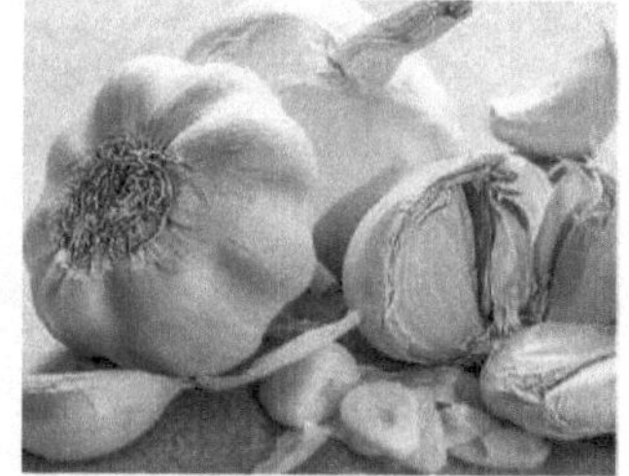

116. Microwave a head of garlic for 10 seconds to remove the outer skin easily.

117. Add a small teaspoon of Dijon mustard to macaroni and cheese to give it a twist.

118. Prevent minced garlic from burning by adding 4 tablespoons of water to the garlic before adding the oil. Cook until the water evaporates, and then add oil to continue to sauté.

119. If onion or garlic begin to sprout, they're not bad. You can still use them – just don't eat the sprouted part; it's bitter.

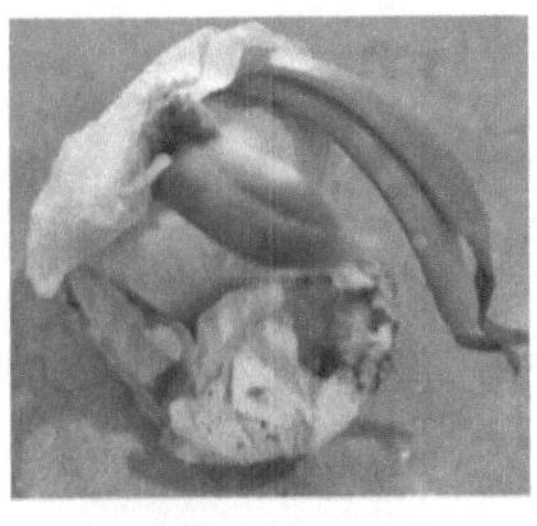

Picture by C.A. Simonson

120. For fluffier rice, place the uncooked rice in a sieve and run under cold water until it runs clear. (This doesn't work with instant rice).

121. Use cheddar cheese soup for easy macaroni and cheese. Boil your own noodles until done, and then add the undiluted soup. Add variety with hamburger or salsa.

122.　Make spaghetti easier to eat for little ones by chopping up pasta noodles.

123.　Don't add salt to water for cooking pasta until it starts to boil. If you add it at the beginning, it can settle to the bottom and make small pits in your pan. It will also take the water longer to boil.　-Pat Everwine/IN

124.　Ladle a little of the water pasta was boiled into the spaghetti sauce to infuse rich flavor.

125.　Keep pasta from sticking together by adding a tablespoon or two of spaghetti sauce – to the water it's boiled in. Adding oil keeps it from sticking together but will not allow the sauce to stick to the pasta.

My new husband couldn't figure why his baked potato had so much grit in it. As a young married woman, I wasn't taught that potatoes needed to be washed before baking. Who knew? I learned quick when I heard him chewing sand!

SOUPS &

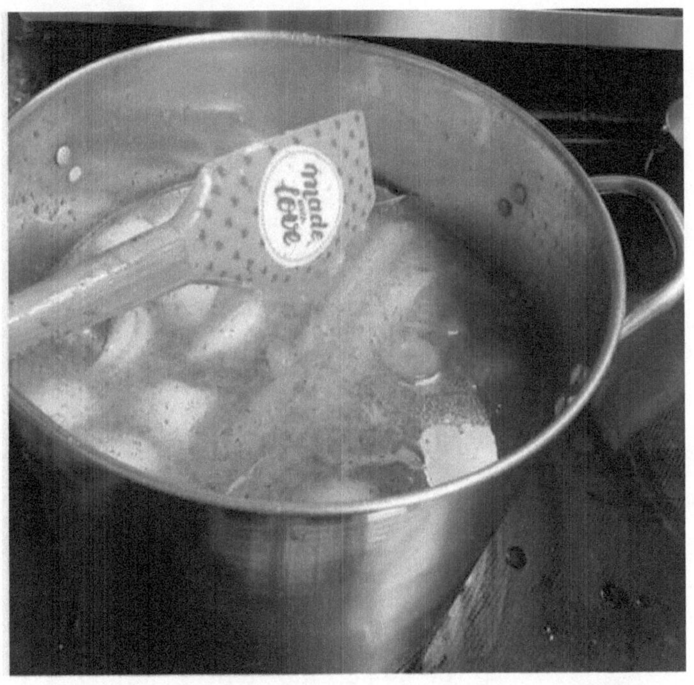

-Bone broth soup - Picture by Terri Lee - Colorado

SAUCES

DID YOU KNOW?

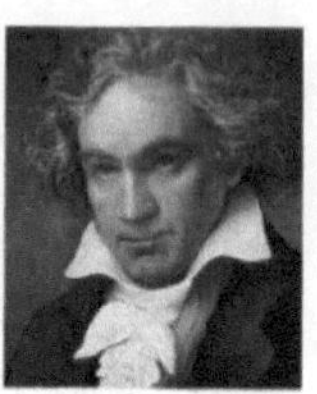

Ludwig van Beethoven said,

"Only the pure of heart can make good soup."

Soup was first mentioned in the Bible when Esau traded his birthright for a bowl of lentil stew. (Genesis 25:34)

"Watch out for the 'Esau syndrome' – trading away God's lifelong gift in order to satisfy a short-term appetite."

(Hebrews 12:16-17- *The Message*)

✠

Portable soup was devised in the 18th century by boiling seasoned meat until a thick, resinous syrup was left that could be dried and stored for months at a time.

How do you make soup richer? Add 24 carrots.

✠

Campbell's soup with its invention in 1897, sold for 10 cents a can boasting 21 varieties. Today, with hundreds of varieties, Americans consume 2.5 billion cans of Campbell's soup each year.

SOUPS

126. Bone broth is a big trend that's healthy and 'skinny' at the same time. Make your own! Save bones from ham or beef (or even steaks) and boil them. You have instant bone broth that's healthy and tasty (with no preservatives).

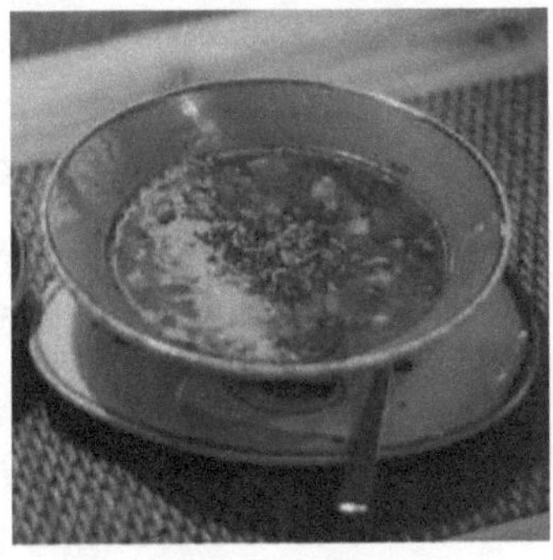

127. Skim any foam that rises to the top both when you're making your stock and when you've added your soup ingredients. This guarantees a clear broth.

128. Instant potatoes are a good soup thickener.

129. If soup becomes too fatty, drop an ice cube in it. The fat will congeal and rise to the top where you can remove it.

130. Add two stalks of celery cut in chunks to your bean soup to make it easier to digest.

131. Soup too bland? Add Worcestershire sauce, soy sauce, or citrus juice. A little tomato paste will also improve flavors.

132. If stew is over-seasoned with garlic, add a cloth bag of parsley. It will absorb the garlic taste.

133. Drop a leaf of lettuce into a pot of soup to absorb the extra grease. Remove the lettuce and throw away.

134. Sauté vegetables such as onions and celery in butter before adding broth and other vegetables to the soup mix. It brings out the rich flavors.

135. My Aunt Laura was known for her delicious fresh tomato soup (tomatoes and milk only). She put a pinch of baking soda into her soup so that it would not curdle.

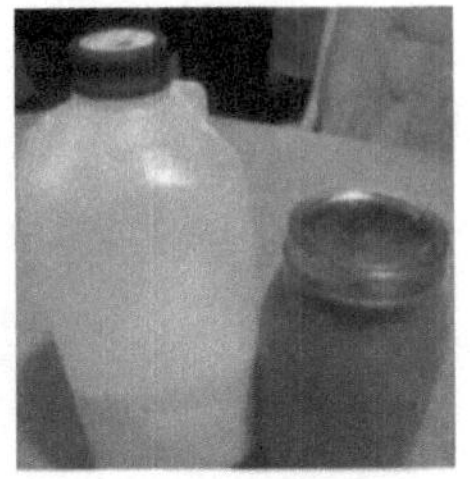

Picture by C.A. Simonson

136. Soup too salty? Add a whole pared potato. It will absorb the salt. Discard the potato.

137. For a spicier-tasting tomato soup, add 1 cup of milk (or cream) to 1 cup of spaghetti sauce of your choice.

138. For "free" vegetable soup, save any left-over cooked veggies in the freezer. When there's enough, add tomato juice and seasoning for a quick vegetable soup.

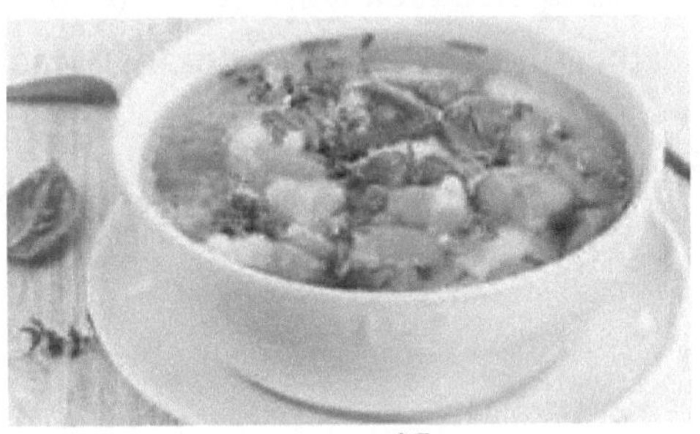

139.   Keep food scraps? Saving carrot ends, potato skins, and other veggies 'throw-aways' can save you on vegetable stock. Save them in the freezer, and when you have enough, boil them in water with seasonings. Throw away the cooked skins and pieces, strain the broth, and you end up with a flavorful vegetable soup stock.

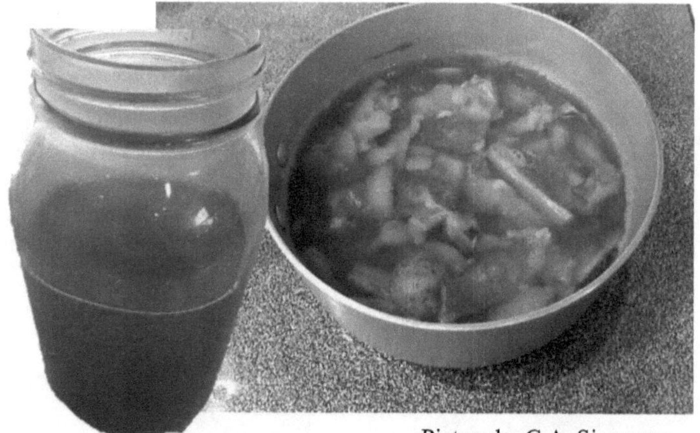

Picture by C.A. Simonson

140.   Vegetable stock is a good soup base for any soup.Add a little cooking wine or vinegar to get a tangier taste in homemade dressings or condiments.

141. Spaghetti sauce too acidic (tangy)? Add sugar to sweeten, or a teaspoon of baking soda until desired taste is achieved. Too sweet? Add more vinegar.

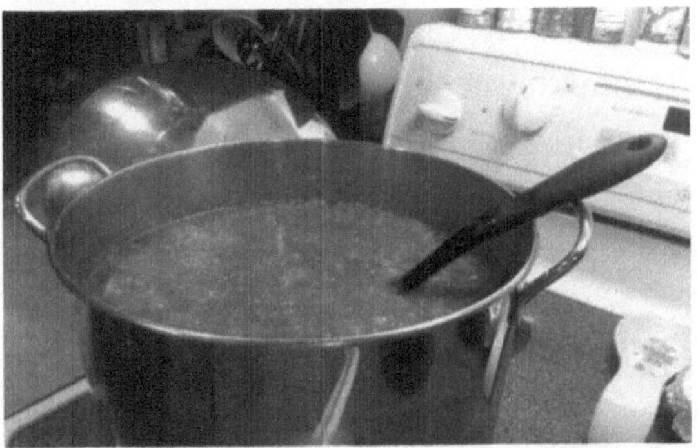

Picture by C.A. Simonson

142. For a tangy-sweet taste, mix ketchup to the sauce.

143. Lower sodium in your homemade soup by using sodium free canned stock (or make your own stock), fresh or frozen vegetables instead of canned.

144. For quick and easy dumplings, use store-bought biscuit dough and drop into soup.

145. For a tasty fall pumpkin soup, use 1 can (2 cups) pumpkin puree, ½ c. brown sugar, and 2 tsp. pumpkin pie spice, and ½ tsp. salt. Add cream to your preference of thickness for soup. (Do not add eggs). Sprinkle pepitas (pumpkin seeds) on top for garnish and crunch!

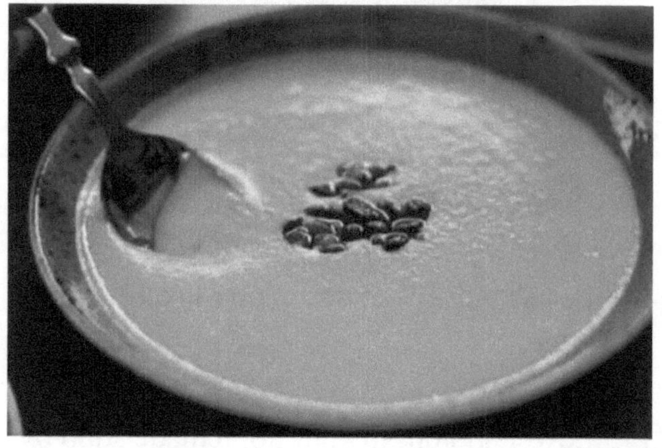

146. Puree butternut squash with pumpkin and use a sweet cream to get that Panera touch on their autumn soup.

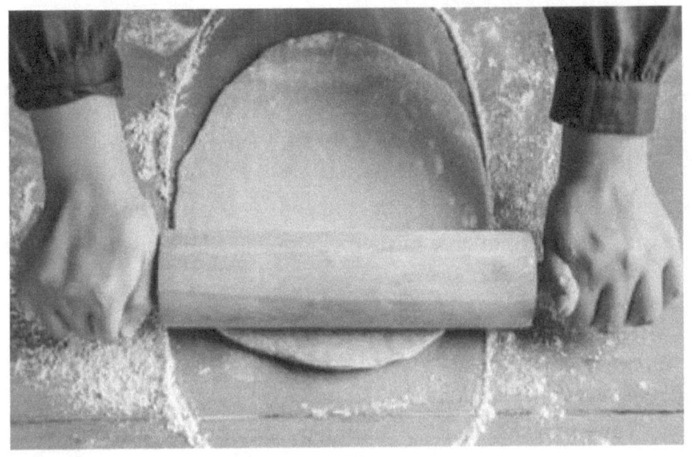

Breads

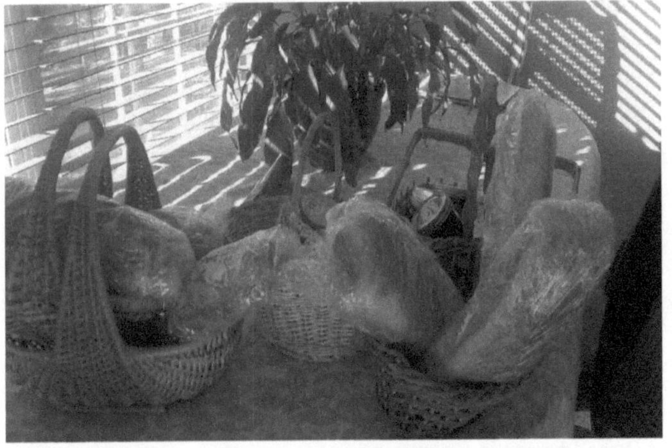

DID YOU KNOW?

Bread has great religious significance associated with communion and 'breaking bread together.' Because of that, it was thought to be a sin to throw away unwanted bread; if you do, it's said you'll go hungry. This could be the reason a lot of people give birds their stale or unwanted bread.

✠

A myth is that bread baked on Good Friday or on Christmas has special healing powers and should be kept throughout the year to ward off sickness. (A good reason to freeze it or make croutons)?

✠

John Montagu, the 4th Earl of Sandwich and a rich gentleman wanted a convenient way to eat his meat while on the go. It is said he asked his servant to bring him meat stuffed between two slices of bread so that he could eat while doing other things. Apparently, his friends took notice and asked for 'the same as Sandwich.' And so, the name stuck.

✠

The inner part of the bread encased by the crust is called the "crumb." That is why small bits of this part of the bread are called crumbs.

BREADS

148. Make your own self-rising flour with 4 cups of flour, 2 teaspoons of salt, and 2 teaspoons of baking powder. Store in tightly covered container.

149. Hot water kills yeast. Make sure the water is lukewarm by touching your wrist.

150. For a shiny bread crust, brush with one egg white beaten with 1 tablespoon water before baking.

151. A tip from my mother:
For a softer crust, brush milk over the dough before baking and melted butter or margarine over the crust immediately after baking. For a crisper crust, brush loaves with water and mist a couple times during baking.

152. For a finer texture of homemade bread, use milk instead of water.

153. For fluffier bread, add 2 beaten eggs to the dough.

154. To slice warm, fresh bread more easily, set it on its side.

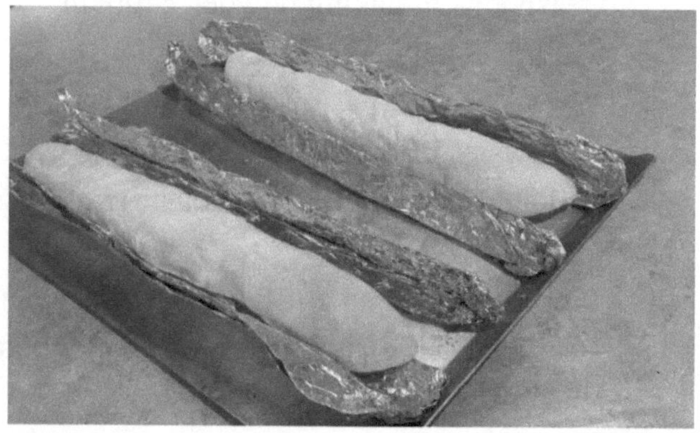

Picture by C.A. Simonson

155. No French or Italian bread pans for long rolls? Make your own with aluminum foil to keep the dough from going flat.

156. Spray butter spray (or butter-flavored oil) on top of buns and pop in the oven at 350 degrees for a few minutes for a golden glaze and crisp top.

157. Shortening is better for greasing pans than spray oil or butter as it doesn't absorb into the dough.

158. Hands too sticky when working with dough? Dust with flour if kneading bread. Oil with butter or vegetable oil if working with biscuits.

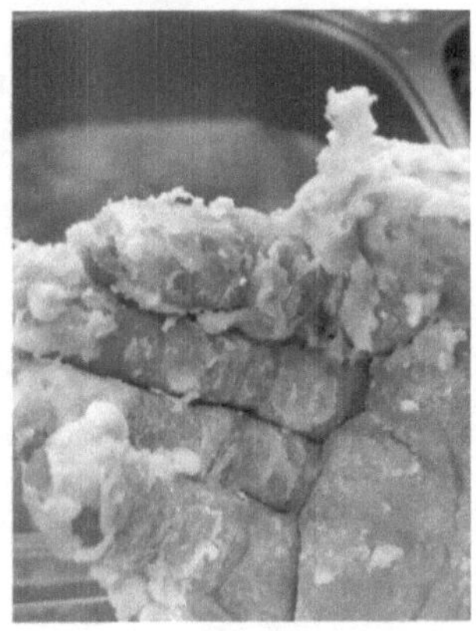

159. How to get that sticky goo off your hands? Let them dry a bit, then briskly rub your hands together over the waste basket. Rinse with cool water. (Hot water makes them even stickier).

160. Knead the dough for 30 seconds to improve the texture of baking powder biscuits.

161. For fluffiest baking powder biscuits or shortcake, make sure your baking powder is fresh (no older than 6 months).

162. Make muffins better by sprinkling raw sugar on top before baking. It gives a crusty, sweet topping.

163. Muffins or biscuits may be too dry if the oven is too hot, or if you've handled them too much in preparation.

164. For the best quick bread, be careful not to overmix the dough. Mix only until combined.

165. Nut breads have better flavor if stored 24 hours before serving.

166. Bread dough can be frozen. Flatten thin so that it defrosts faster. Butter the tops of rolls before freezing dough to keep them from drying out.

167. Spread bread with butter, Mayo or topping before adding tomatoes or meat to prevent soggy sandwiches.

168.   Make your own garlicky croutons by cubing old bread. Slice off the crust, roll bread cubes in olive oil, dust with garlic powder/salt and bake in a low oven until light brown.

169.   Add a teaspoon of instant potatoes to your pancake mixture to make lighter pancakes.

170.   Add ½ tsp. baking soda to your waffle/pancake mix for fluffy pancakes.

171.   Make your own fruity pancake/waffle syrup by thinning your favorite jam with little water. Bring to a boil.

172.   Crepes aren't hard to make – just thin the pancake batter with milk. Skinny pancakes (less calories) with fruit compote or fruit jam wrapped inside make a wonderful breakfast!

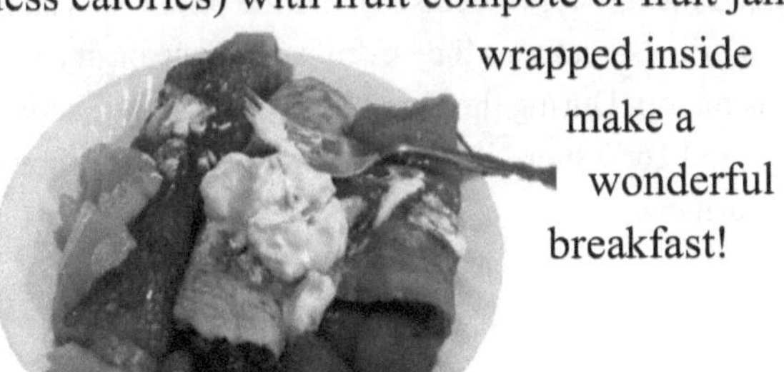

Picture by C.A. Simonson

Food had power in the old mythic tradition...

In New Mexico during winter months, children sometimes appeared in classrooms with a large clove of garlic strung on a string around the neck. It was supposed to drive away sickness (and evil spirits).

☩

Ginger was considered the herb of paradise. In the Far East in ancient times, it was thought to bring one closer to Deity. It was linked with the solar fire, as was cinnamon. It was one of the key ingredients of magical practices, including love-lore.

☩

In China in times past, leftover rice could not be discarded, for it was sacred to the Chinese god of thunder.

☩

In medieval times, mince pies were made with real minced meat (beef or venison) and the pastry was shaped like a crib. Sometimes they even had a little pastry infant Jesus on top. During the Commonwealth period between 1640 and 1660 such 'idolatrous' practices were banned by the Puritans.

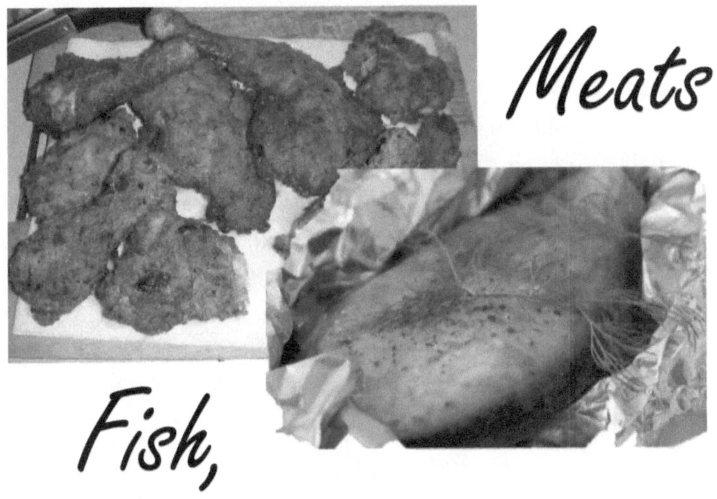

Meats

Fish,

Game & Poultry

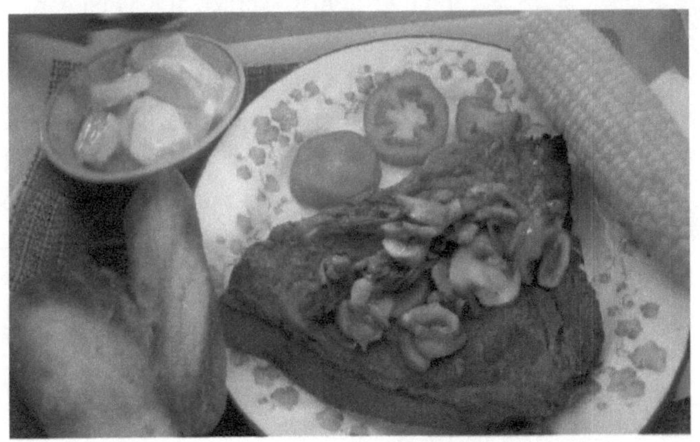

Picture by C.A. Simonson

DID YOU KNOW?

An old story goes that the newlywed bride cut her beef in half before roasting it. When asked why, she said because her mother did it that way, and it was the best roast ever. Asking her mother why she did it, she was told, "Because that's the way Grandma always did it. It was always the best roast ever!"

Grandma was finally asked why she cut her meat in two pieces before roasting it. She replied. "It was the only way it fit in my pan."

✠

~Cornflakes makes a wonderful crunchy breading! And they were discovered by accident.

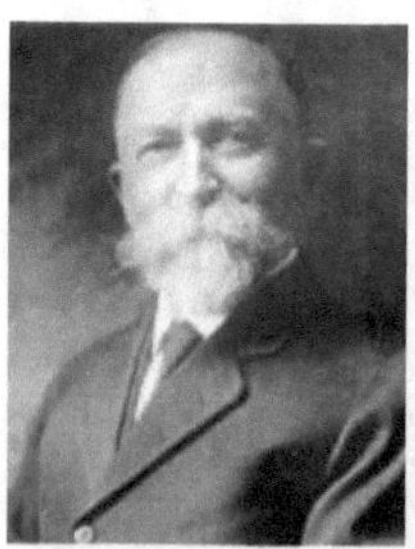

Dr. John Kellogg, a medical doctor and nutritionist, worked at a Michigan sanitarium run by Seventh-Day Adventists in the 1890s. He and his brother, Will, needed to create a more easily digestible form of bread for patients. *History Today* reports that they overboiled their wheat by mistake and, rather than dough, it formed into dry flakes. It was surprisingly tasty, and they decided to go ahead and feed it to patients anyway. It was liked so much, they perfected their experiment. They toasted maize in 1898 and the first 'corn flakes' were created!

MEATS, FISH, GAME & POULTRY

BEEF

173. Adding salt to meat before cooking prevents it from browning. Wait to salt meat midway through, or until it's done.

174. Rotate your roasting meat half-way through the baking process to get all sides evenly roasted.

175. Make sure your pan is piping hot before adding the meat to sear. If you have a metal roasting pan (or crockpot pan), you can sear the meat directly in that pan.

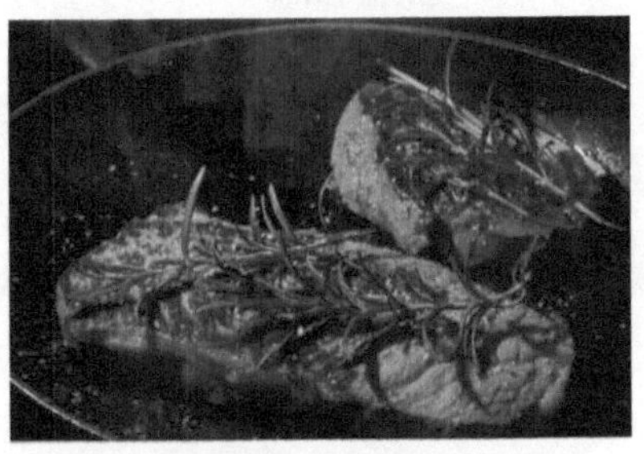

176. Sear roast beef on each side in olive oil before putting in the oven or crockpot.

This seals in the juices. (Works with steaks also).

177. A roast with a bone roasts twice as fast as one without a bone. Why? Because the bone acts as a conductor.

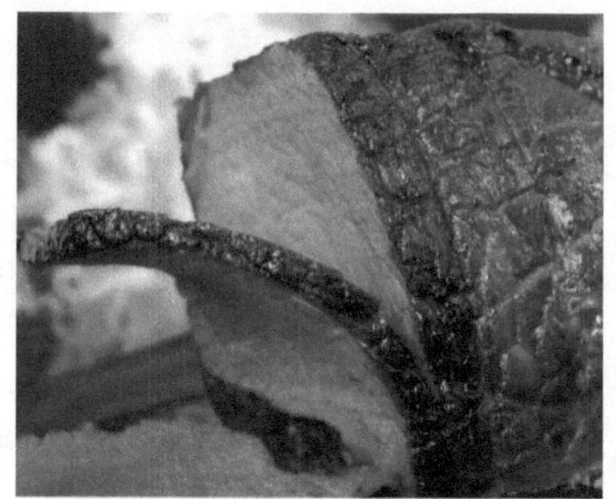

178. Sprinkle dry beef gravy mix or dry onion soup mix over a roast before putting in the oven or crockpot for great flavor and glaze. – Susie Adams/MO

179. Add tomatoes to a tougher cut of roast beef (like chuck or arm roast) to help tenderize it.

180. Cook with kosher salt; season with sea salt to pull out the flavors in foods.

181.   Add garlic immediately to the recipe if you want a light taste of garlic. Add it at the end of the recipe if you want a stronger taste of garlic.

182.   Slice meat **against the grain** to avoid it being 'chewy.'

183.   Don't throw away the little bit of roast and veggies. Add more water or beef stock to the broth, break up the meat and veggies and make stew! Need to stretch it? Add beans, lentils, barley, or noodles.

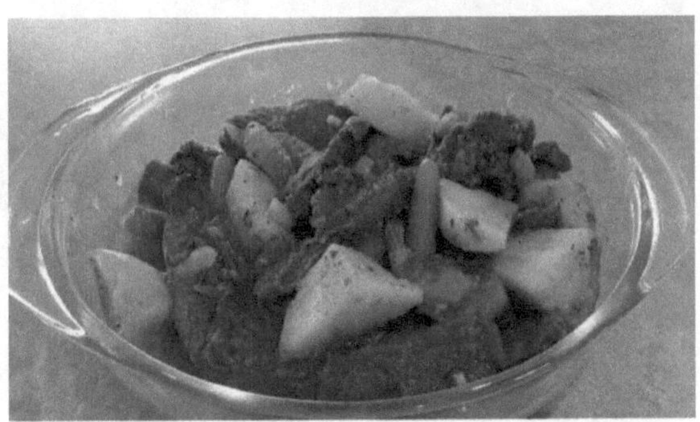

Picture by C.A. Simonson

184.   Frozen steaks taste better than thawed steaks because they lose less moisture and cook more evenly.

185. For evenly-sliced pieces of meat for stir-fry, slice the meat into strips while partially frozen.

186. Score your meat (make a crisscross pattern with a knife) before you cook it to absorb marinades and to prevent skin from shrinking away while cooking.

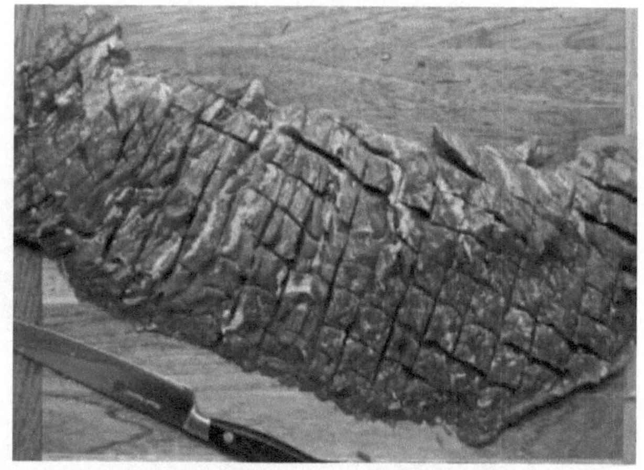

187. If gravy separates, add a pinch of baking soda to get oils and fats to stick back together.

188. For rich brown gravy, add a cup of cold coffee into the gravy mix.

189. For succulent beef gravy, put onion soup mix on the bottom of the roaster. After removing the roast, add one can of creamed soup for a rich brown gravy.

190. Keep lumps out of gravy by mixing the cornstarch (or flour) with cold water first. Then add it to the juices and fats to combine. Use a whisk to keep stirring.

191. For more flavorful hamburgers, add a little minced onion (or dry onion flakes) and no-salt seasoning to raw hamburger. Mix together well and then make into patties.

192. For a juicier hamburger, add a teaspoon of water when frying. It pulls the grease away from the hamburger.

193. Add salsa to your sloppy joes for a tangier taste.

194. Make a tastier meatloaf by combining sausage or other ground meat (such as venison or turkey) to hamburger mix.

195. Oatmeal or saltine crackers can replace breadcrumbs in a meatloaf but be cautious not to add too much. It can also make it dry.

FISH & SEAFOOD

196. If seafood smells fishy, it has started to decay. Throw it out.

197. Take the 'fishy' taste out of salmon or tilapia by removing the brown strip down the middle first.

198. Double-coat fish when breading for a good, crispy layer. Mix your breading, dip meat in an egg wash (egg beaten together with a little water), dip in breading, and repeat.

199. Swab each side of raw salmon with milk and store, covered, in the refrigerator overnight to reduce odor, enhance the flavor, and maintain its color.

200. Tenderize fish by defrosting it in milk.

201. Boil raw shrimp with caraway seed for a better flavor. Make sure water comes to a boil before adding frozen shrimp. Remove once they become pink to prevent mushiness.

202. Change your breading varieties: add crushed corn

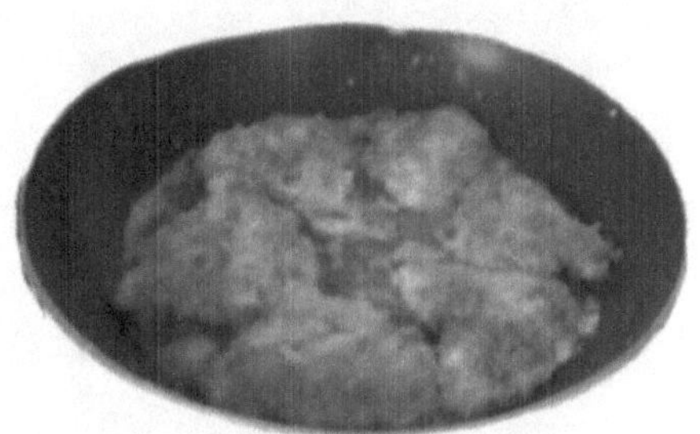

Picture by C.A. Simonson

flakes or potato chips to your flour and/or Panko® bread crumbs.

CHICKEN/ TURKEY/DUCK

203. Chicken thighs are more flavorful, juicier, and cheaper than chicken breasts – and cook in half the time.

204. Save the broth after roasting chicken or beef. It makes a great soup base. It can be frozen for up to six months.

205. Shred cooked chicken quickly with a hand mixer or food processor.

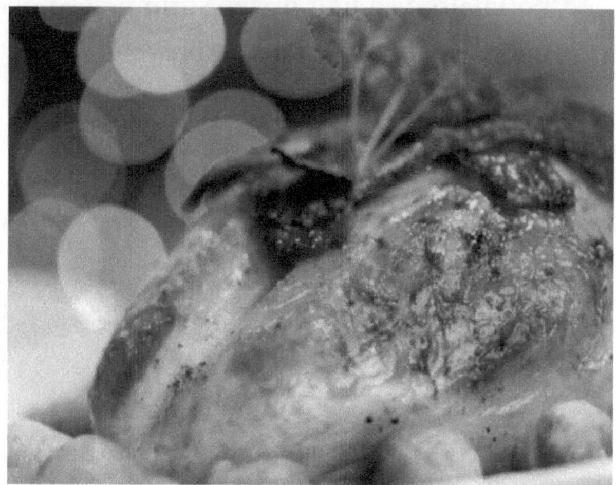

206. When stewing chicken, cool in the broth before shredding or cubing it. It will have twice the flavor.

207. For a wonderful, different flavor of roast turkey, stuff the turkey with wedges of lemons, limes, and oranges. A subtle citrus flavor emerges.

208. For a moister turkey, remove the legs and wings and cook them wrapped in foil separately.

209. Use crushed potato or veggie chips as a topping for baked chicken pot pie instead of pie crust.

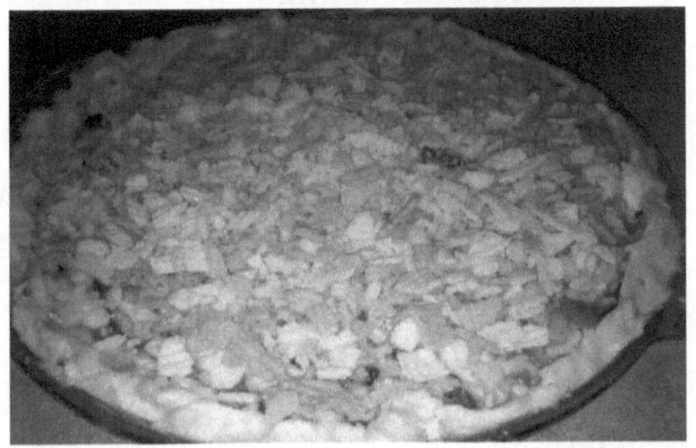

Picture by C.A. Simonson

210. For a quick and easy chicken casserole, eliminate the crust. Mix one can of canned chicken, one can of creamed soup, and one can of Veg-All® veggies. Top with potato chips and heat in oven.

211. Use up or freeze leftover chicken or turkey for pot pie or soup.

PORK

212. Soak bacon in cold water for a few
      minutes before frying in the skillet. This
      lessens the tendency to shrink or curl.

213. Avoid splattering bacon by baking! Put
      bacon on a foil-lined baking pan and bake
      in a preheated oven at 400 degrees for 10-
      12 minutes.

214. Add a pinch of ginger and honey to orange
      juice for a tangy-sweet marinade for
      meats.

215. Cover oranges, apples, pineapple with
      water; add cinnamon and cloves and
      simmer on the stove for a wonderful
      holiday aroma.

216. Use this same combination as a tasty glaze
      on ham or pork chops.

217. For a very moist ham, empty a can of
      Coke into the baking pan. Wrap the ham in
      aluminum foil and bake. Thirty minutes
      before it's finished, remove the foil and

allow the drippings to mix with the Coke for a wonderful brown gravy.

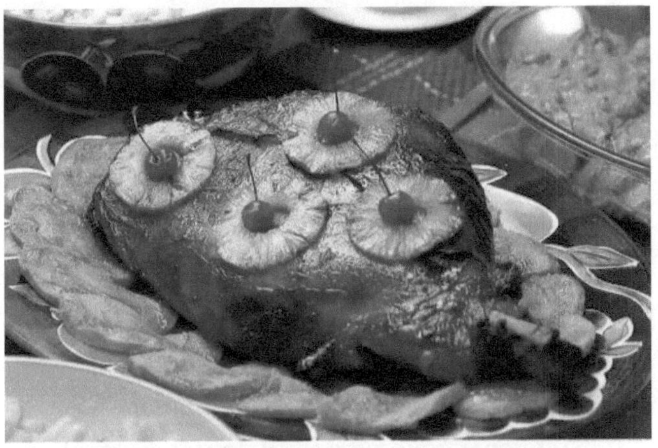

218. Add Dijon mustard to pineapple juice to spread over ham while it's baking.

219. Adding pineapple rings and juice to a ham not only keeps it moist and adds flavor, but also tenderizes it.

WILD GAME

DUCK

220. Use pickling spices wrapped in cheesecloth and set it alongside a wild duck for succulent flavor! If no cheesecloth is handy, a clean baby sock works (according to my mother).

WILD TURKEY

221. Wild turkey becomes more tender and juicier if covered completely with chicken stock and cooked in a crockpot several hours on low. *(Use only the breast).

VENISON

222. Many people dislike deer meat because of the filmy coating it can leave in the mouth. This comes from the deer fat. To keep the "tallow taste" from venison, remove as much fat and any 'white' from the meat before cooking.

223. De-boning deer meat before cooking also helps remove that filmy feeling in the mouth.

224. Soak venison in milk to take the "deer" taste out.

-Jeannie Snell/MO

225. To make a more tender venison, pound the meat and add a little meat tenderizer before cooking.

226. Deer meat will taste different according to what the deer has eaten. If he feeds on nuts, berries, weeds, the flavor may be strong (gamey); but if he feeds on corn, you won't be able to tell the difference between deer and beef.

227. If steaks or chops are too thin, make them even

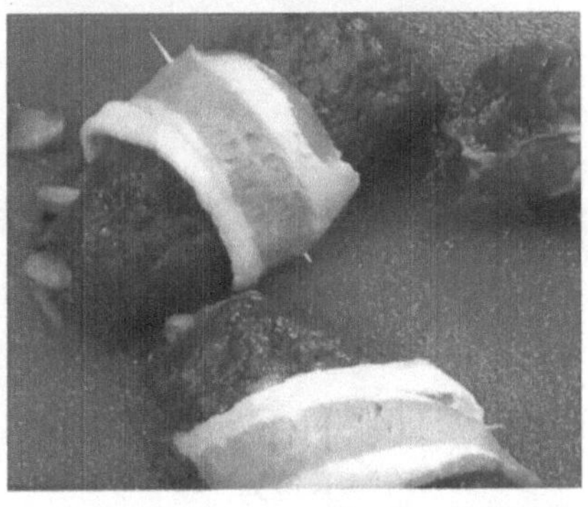

Venison Roll-ups
-Picture by C.A. Simonson

thinner by pounding them first. Stuff them with mushrooms and/or onion and roll up. Secure with a strip of bacon and a toothpick. Roast, grill, or fry as usual.

BEANS

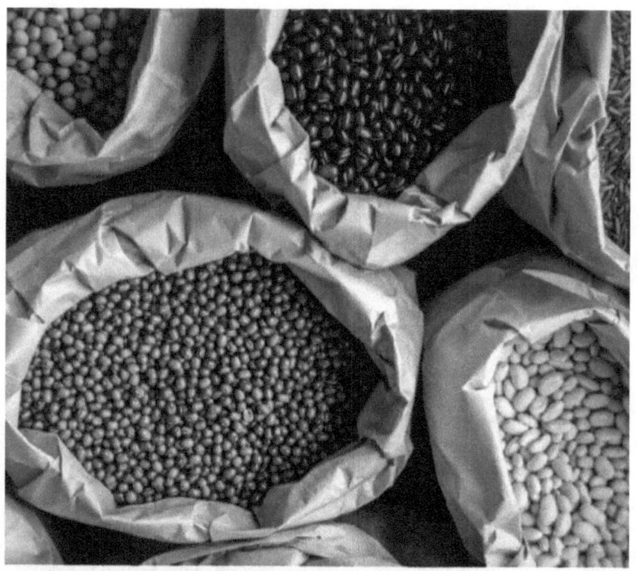

228.　Soaking dry beans overnight in salted water helps to eliminate gassiness, but also ensures the bean remains creamy inside, not mealy.

229.   For great-tasting baked beans, add molasses to your brown sugar mixture.

230.   Eliminate the gas side effects of beans by adding a dash of baking soda while cooking.

231.   Beans may foam while cooking. This is normal and won't affect taste. To eliminate foam, add a tsp. of butter or oil.

232.   Make a quick bean soup with leftover ham pieces. Add a can each of butter beans, kidney beans, pinto beans, (or any others you like) and a can of tomato sauce. No need to salt – the ham does the work.

233.   Buying dried beans may be more work, but they are almost three times cheaper and have less sodium and preservatives.

234.   Simmer – don't boil beans. Cook on low heat for several hours, remembering to stir often. More water may be needed as they expand.

YOUR FOOD HACKS:

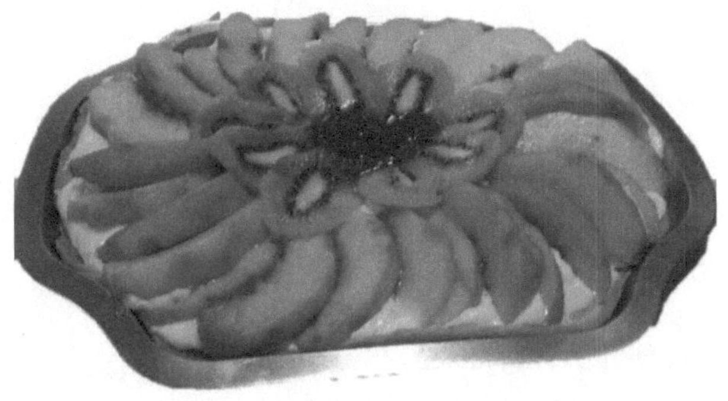

Desserts

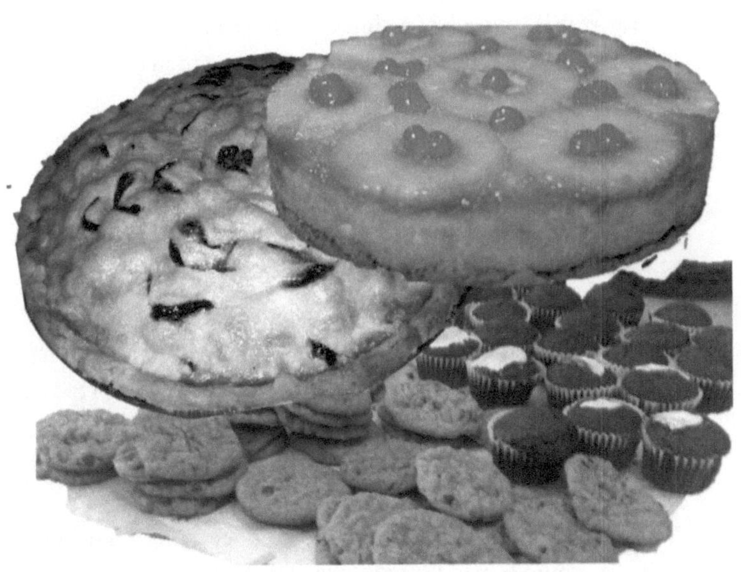

Pictures by C.A. Simonson

DID YOU KNOW?

Did the Pilgrims eat pumpkin pie? In a way, they did. In 1621, there were no ovens for baking. Sugar had dwindled, but their Indian friends showed them how to fix a dish called "pompion," which was stewed pumpkin. They sliced off the 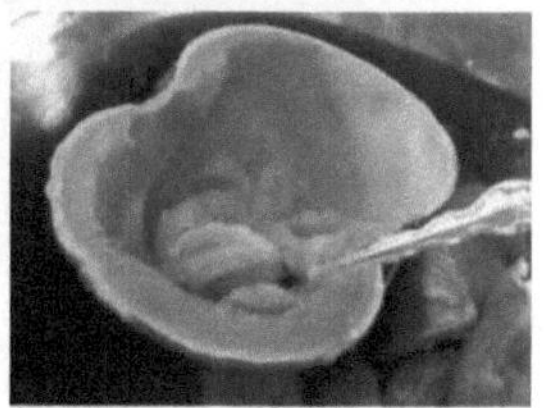 pumpkin top, removed the seeds and strings, and filled the insides with milk and honey. The pumpkin was then put in the hot ashes to bake. They may not have eaten a real pumpkin pie, but what they had was pumpkin pudding without the crust.

During WWII, sugar was rationed -to the detriment of many desserts. The government encouraged people to mash and freeze carrots and use the sweet veggie in other desserts. Having many cans of canned carrots after the war, culinary chefs came up with the idea of carrot cake.

In the late 1800s, ice cream was served in glass containers only large enough to have a lick or two. Called "penny licks," customers licked the glass clean and returned it to the vendor. Without washing it, the next customer was served. Due to the spread of tuberculosis at that time, penny licks were banned in 1899 Another method had to be found. A dessert chef came up with the waffle cone in the early 1900s when created with a crisp, curled waffle like container to hold ice cream. It debuted at the St. Louis World Fair in 1904. The first "ice cream cone."

DESSERTS

235. Preheat any baking pans, cookie sheets, muffin tins, etc. for better results when baking.

236. To cream butter and sugar faster, rinse your bowl with hot water.

237. Before melting chocolate, grease the pan first so it doesn't stick.

238. Use the same measuring cup that you beat your eggs in to measure shortening or peanut butter. It will slip right out without sticking to the sides.

239. Brown sugar too hard? Put a few marshmallows in the bag.

CAKE

240. Keep cakes or brownies from sticking to the pan by dusting the pan first. Coat the bottom and sides with enough shortening to make it shiny. Put a little flour in the pan and move it from side to side until all parts are "dusted." Dispose of the extra flour.

241. Add extra moistness to a store-bought cake mix by adding two extra egg yolks.

242. Does your cake seem heavy or dense? Not as light as you wish? Make sure to cream together the shortening and sugar well before adding the eggs.

243. Add margarine or butter in place of oil to a cake mix to get a richer flavor.

244. Add a box of instant pudding to any box cake mix for richer flavor and moistness.

245. Add milk to a box mix rather than water to add extra flavor and density to your cake.

246. For a darker, richer-looking chocolate cake, add 1 tsp. baking soda to the other dry ingredients.

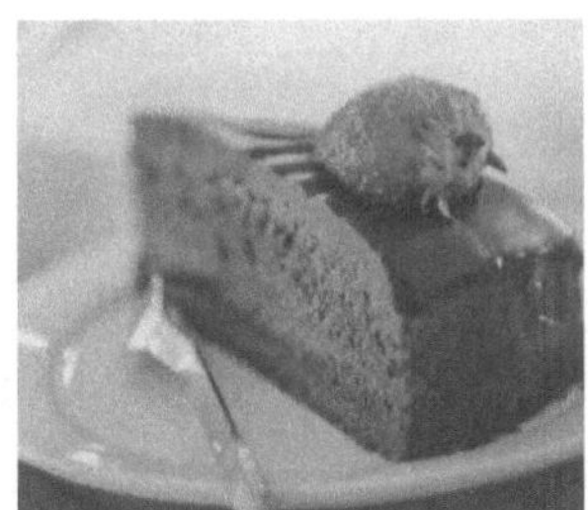

247. Add two teaspoons of almond flavoring to a white cake box mix to give flavor; also add it to the frosting.

248. Mix a box mix with 1 cup water and 1 cup either pumpkin or applesauce. Tastes like homemade!! Janis Ericksen/S.D.

249. Applesauce is a substitute for eggs (1 cup to 2 eggs) for eggless cake!

250. Double the amount of canned frosting by whipping it with your mixer. (It also means fewer calories and sugar per serving).

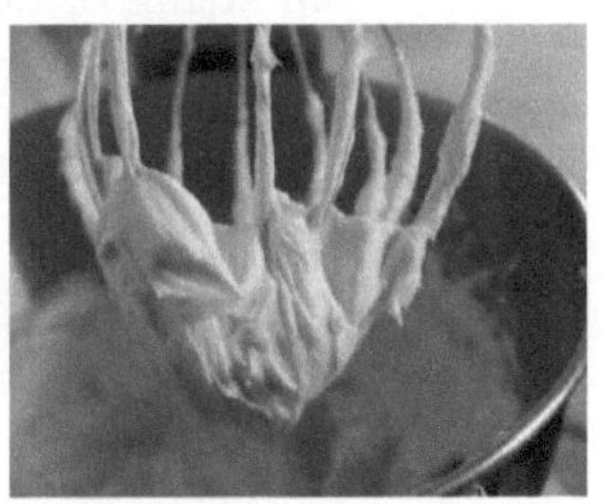

251. Use margarine (or butter) instead of oil in your cake mix for a richer, tastier cake.

252.   Make too much frosting? Save it in the refrigerator for up to a month.

253.   Want to frost a flat top on your round cake? Cut off the mound and turn the cake upside down so you frost the bottom.

254.   Keep the frosting from dripping off the cake by sprinkling the cake with powdered sugar first.

255.   When using a box cake mix, add a snack cup of pudding to make it extra moist.
-Krystal Heimsoth/MO

256.   If you must cut a warm cake, use a piece of string or dental floss instead of a knife.

257.   A cake is done if the sides pull away slightly from the cake pan, or springs back when touched lightly by your finger.

COOKIES

258. Cookies made with room temperature butter will be chewier than if made with cold butter.

259. Room temperature eggs make cookies fluffier in texture.

260. Mouth-watering, tender cookies come from less flour. Be careful not to pack the flour in the measuring cup.

261. Want a butterier flavor in your cookies? Chill the dough for a few hours first.

262. Rolled cookie dough works much better when it's cooled overnight first.

263. Add lemon extract instead of vanilla to sugar cookies for a fresh new taste.

264. Dip cookie cutters in flour and shake off excess for easier cutting.

265.   Bake cookies directly on parchment paper for a breeze of a cleanup.

266.   When making cake-like, thicker cookies, turn the oven down by 25 degrees to keep the outside from over-baking.

267.   Keep your cookies chewy and moist by storing an apple wedge in the container.

268.   Use the bottom of an empty spool of thread or decorative glass container bottoms for pretty designs in molded cookies.

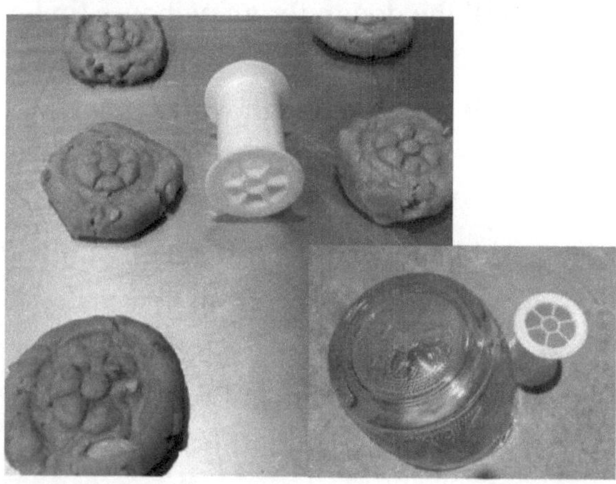

Pictures by C.A. Simonson

269. Instead of folding nuts into brownie batter, sprinkle on top to keep nuts crunchier.

270. Are cookies getting hard? Put a piece of dry bread in with the container.

271. To make cookie "tubes" for filling, wrap warm cookies around a wooden spoon and allow to cool.

272. For crispy, nutty chocolate chip cookies, add 1 cup of Old Fashioned Quaker oatmeal® along with 3-4 crumbled Mr. Goodbar® candy bars to the recipe.

273. No chocolate chips? Break up a candy bar or chunk of chocolate.

274. Unbaked cookie dough can be kept in the freezer for up to nine months.

275. Bake brownies in a glass or shiny tin pan. The bottom gets soggy in a nonstick coated pan.

276.   Sprinkle a little salt on top of brownie
        batter to bring out a chocolatey flavor.

PIE

277.   For flakier pie crust, add an egg yolk and
        enough milk to equal 2/3 cup to 2 ½ cups
        of flour, ½ cup shortening, and ½ cup of
        margarine. Makes two full pie crusts.
        (Save the egg white to brush on top crust
        *Thanks to my mother-in-law for this tip).

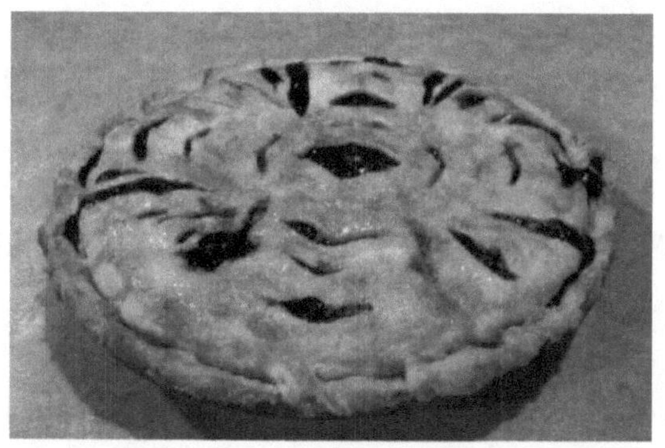

Picture by C.A. Simonson

*Why is it that a guest or your husband
always finds the pits in the pie?*

278. Brush a beaten egg white on top of an uncooked pie crust and then sprinkle with sugar to get a golden, sugary top.

279. Use all brown sugar to get a deeper brown color to your pumpkin pie.

280. Pumpkin or custard-type pies are done when the middle is slightly jiggly. Insert a toothpick in the center. If it comes out without any liquid, it is done.

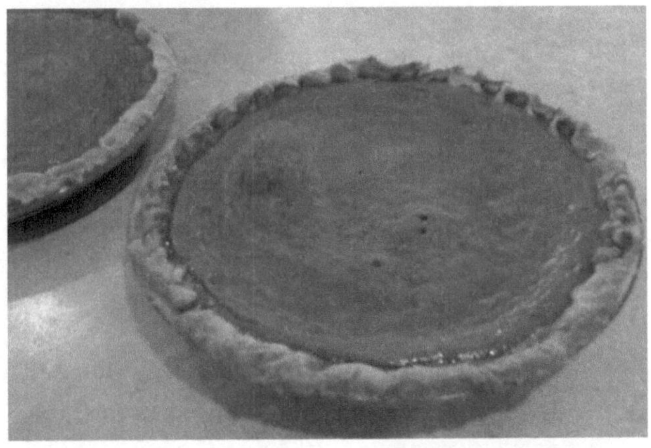

Picture by C.A. Simonson

281. Freeze leftovers of pumpkin puree (or other fruit filling) in 1-2 cup freezer bags for easy retrieval for future recipes.

282. Prepare your own fresh pumpkin pie filling! Remove seeds and strings and then roast the whole pumpkin in the oven until tender. Scoop out the contents. Put into a blender or food processor and puree until smooth. Package in 2 cup containers with spices and freeze to make pumpkin pie (or cookies, cake, bread, soup).

283. Use cinnamon candies when making an apple pie or applesauce. -Betty Shortt/ MO

284. Glass pie pans work better than tin. It evenly distributes the heat and makes the bottom of the pie golden brown.

285. Prevent a pie crust from a soggy bottom by sprinkling powdered sugar over the bottom before adding cream or custard filling.

286.   Keep the pie filling from bubbling over by putting the top crust completely over the bottom crust before crimping.

287.   Another way to keep juices from bubbling over is to put tube-shaped pasta, like rigatoni, into the holes in the crust. This allows the steam to escape without the contents spilling out. Remove the pasta and discard when the pie is done.

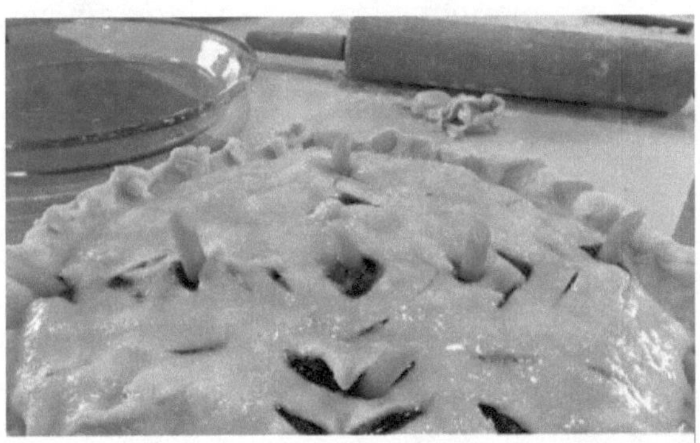

Picture by C.A. Simonson

288.   Put wax paper or parchment paper on the counter before rolling dough for pie or bread. To keep the paper stable from slipping, sprinkle a little water on the counter first. Easy clean-up!

289. To keep a one-crust bottom from bubbling during baking, poke a few holes with a fork in your pie crust bottom before putting in the oven.

290. The fluffiest meringue comes from room-temperature egg whites. To warm eggs, put them in a bowl of warm water.

291. Keep meringue from shrinking on your pie top by spreading to the very edges of the crust.

292. Sweeten tart fruit like blackberries with ½ tsp. of baking soda before adding any sugar.

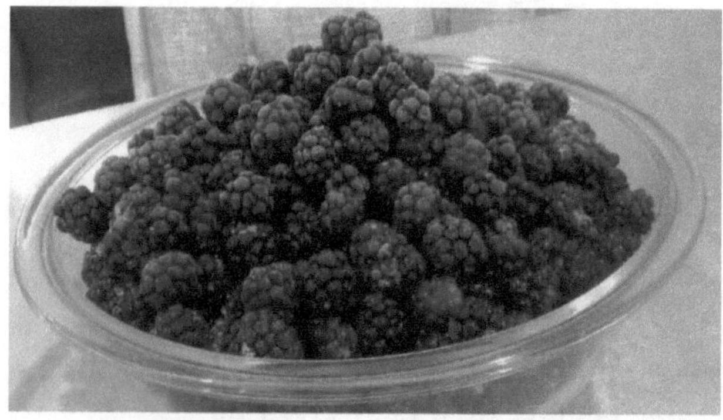

Picture by C.A. Simonson

293. Keep ice cream from getting freezer burn by storing the tub upside down in the freezer.

294. Use parchment paper instead of waxed paper for making high-temperature candy.

295. For creamy homemade fudge, stir in marshmallows before pouring into the pan. They melt immediately and make the fudge smooth.

EASY LAST-MINUTE DESSERTS

296. For a quick and easy dessert, prepare any flavor of cooked pudding and then add a scoop of ice cream into bowls of hot pudding cups.

297. For a quick and *light pineapple cake*, add a can of crushed pineapple (instead of water) to angel food cake and bake as directed.

298. Make *cakebox cookies* when you don't have time for mixing a lot of ingredients. 1 box (any flavor) cake mix plus 2 eggs and ½ cup of oil. Drop on cookie sheet and bake. Lemon cookies are my favorite— dusted with powdered sugar. Add a bit of almond flavoring to vanilla cake mix for almond cookies.

299. Make *pumpkin-spice cookies* with one box of spice cake mix and one can of packed pumpkin. Mix together well and drop by spoonfuls onto a cookie sheet. Bake at 350 degrees.

300. The *3-2-1 mug cake* is easy and fast for one person's sweet tooth – low in calories too. Combine one box of angel food cake mix with another box of cake mix 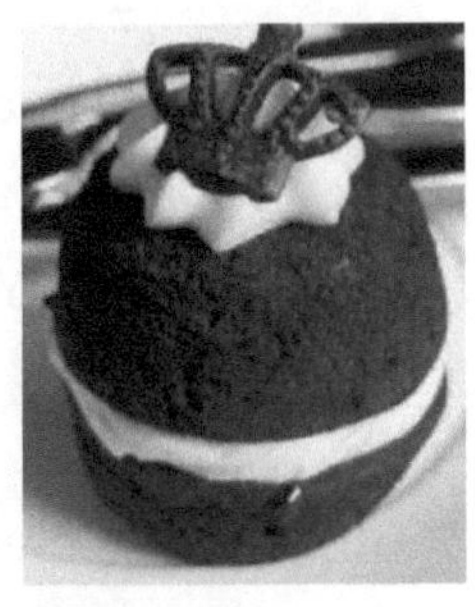 (your choice of flavors). Spray a mug with nonstick cooking spray. Mix 3 level Tablespoons of your cake concoction with 2 Tablespoons of water in the mug. Microwave on high for 1 minute.

301. Freeze whipped orange yogurt for easy *push-ups*. Cut the bottom off the yogurt container; put a popsicle stick into the yogurt. Cover with foil and freeze. When ready to eat, run the container under hot water and slip the push-up out to enjoy.

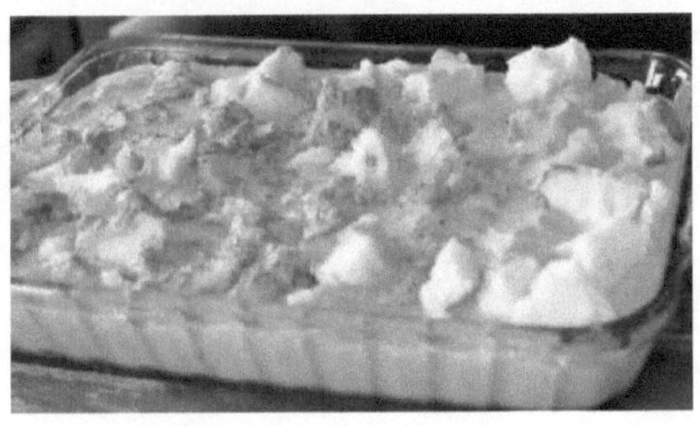

302.   Left-over angel food cake? Tear into chunks and mix into Jell-O®. When partially set, mix with whipped cream for a whole new dessert.

303.   Use crescent roll dough to bake up quickie pies. Piece together two triangles of crescent dough to make a square. Spoon 1-2 tsp of minced apples in the middle. Sprinkle with sugar and cinnamon and bake as usual. Easier yet – use jam for filling.

Beverages

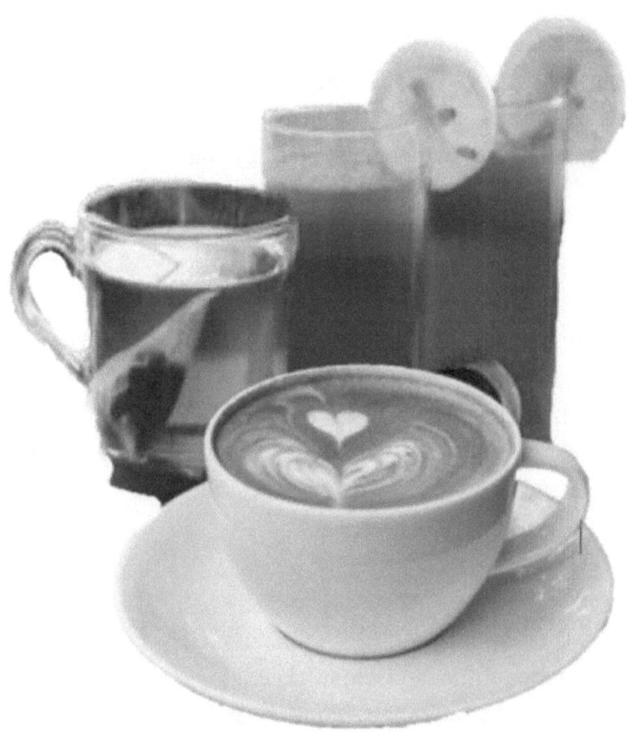

DID YOU KNOW?

Tea bags were invented in America in the early 1800s and were initially used to hold samples of teas brought from India. Today, teabags make 96% of all cups of tea served around the world.

✠

"Ramune" (Japanese for "lemonade") produces its bubbly beverages in wasabi, kimchi, curry and teriyaki flavors, as well as less spicy—but no less unusual—flavors such as bubble gum, white champagne, blueberry and banana.

✠

Before 1908, coffee was brewed with filters made of cloth. If no cloth was available, a sock would do. After getting fed up with coffee's bitter taste caused by cloth filters, German homemaker Melitta Bentz took a page from her son's schoolbook and filtered her coffee through it. She patented her invention, and now we have paper coffee filters.

✠

Coffee was first imported from Arabia to Europe in the 1500s. While people in Christian Europe liked the caffeinated drink, it was greeted with suspicion. Some called it "Satan's drink." Pope Clement VIII (1536-1605) argued that the drink was so good that it would be a "sin" to let only "pagans drink it."

BEVERAGES

304.　Trick yourself into drinking more water by making it flavorful. Add fresh fruit like lemon, lime, oranges, strawberries to a cold pitcher of water and let them infuse the water with flavor.

305.　Freeze nasturtium or violet petals into ice cubes to add beauty to your iced drink.

306.　Keep your large pitchers of fruit juice or lemonade from diluting with ice. Put the ice cubes in a plastic bag first.

307.　Freeze fruit juice or punch into ice cubes to prevent plain ice cubes from diluting the beverage.

308.　Honey does not spoil. Ever. And so good for you. Use it to flavor your beverage.

309.　Add ¼ tsp. baking soda to 8 ounces of citrus juice (orange, lemon, grapefruit, pineapple) to give it fizz and reduce acidity.

310. Put fresh peppermint or spearmint leaves
in your tea for a refreshing mint tea.

311. Add watered-down blackberry
jelly to iced tea for excellent
blackberry tea. No sugar
needed!

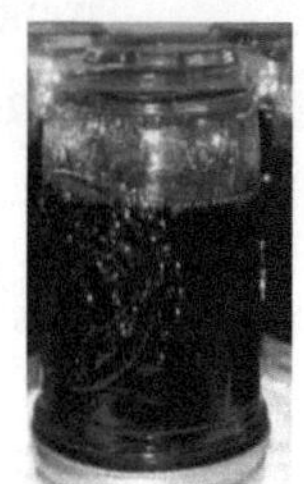

Picture by C.A. Simonson

312. Save the juice
from peaches to
add to tea for peach tea.

313. Dissolve a hard lemon candy drop in hot
tea for lemon tea.

314. Add fresh mint leaves to tea for mint tea.
Or, freeze them in ice cubes.

315. Keep your coffee grounds in the freezer
for fresher tasting coffee.

316. Coffee too bitter? Acidic? Add a pinch of
baking soda.

317. Add flavors to your hot chocolate with cinnamon candies, peppermint candies, or a little vanilla.

318. Like flavored coffee or tea? Melt a few cinnamon or peppermint candies in the cup while brewing your hot beverage. (Works with hot chocolate too).

319. For quick hot chocolate, mix together 2 cups nonfat dry milk powder, 1 cup chocolate drink mix (like Nesquik®), 3/4 cup powdered sugar, and 3/4 cup non-dairy powdered creamer. Store in a covered container. Use 1/4 cup mix with 1 cup of hot water.

320. Frozen fruits generally blend better than fresh fruit. Freeze over-ripe bananas to use in smoothies. The taste is better.

321. Put your liquids in the blender first, and then put your fruit or veggies on top. It makes it easier on the blades and motor.

322. Make too much smoothie?
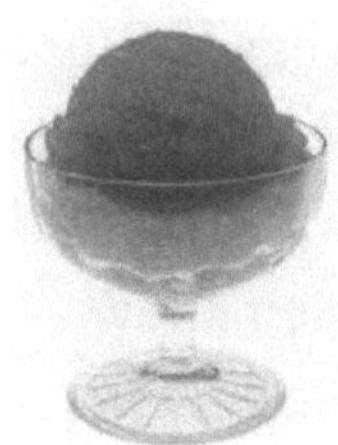Freeze the rest. Mix raspberries, bananas and orange juice for a wonderful sorbet later.

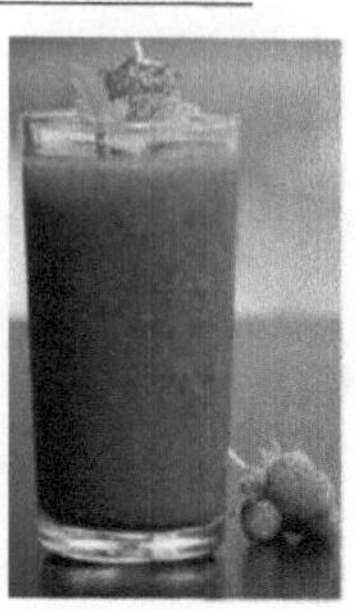

323. If you like avocado, spinach or kale in a smoothie, but can't use them up fast enough, chop and freeze it into ice cubes to be used when you need it.

324. Spinach taste can be masked easily in a smoothie. Get your protein and iron by tossing some spinach in with peanut butter, chocolate syrup and milk. Yummy!

Cooking &

Baking

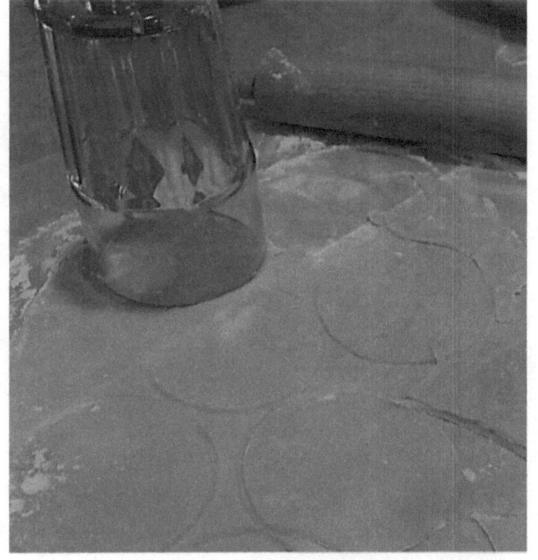

Picture by C.A. Simonson

Hacks

DID YOU KNOW?

Salt was a commodity considered a symbol of honesty and integrity in ages past. A "covenant of salt" was considered a binding agreement thought to last forever. It was used in Bible times. "The Lord God of Israel gave the kingship…to David… by a covenant of salt." (II Chronicles 13:5, NRSV).

✠

The expression "not worth his salt" came from a time around 750 B.C. where slaves were traded for salt.

✠

Soldiers of the Roman Empire (around 500 B.C.) were paid "salt money," (*salarium argentum)*. This is where we get the word "salary."

✠

You may recall "mandrakes" from the Harry Potter movies – a Mediterranean herb that is shaped like a human and supposedly shrieks when being pulled from the ground. Mandrakes (also known as may apples) were used for medicinal and magical purposes and was also used in the Bible. In Genesis 30:14, women believed mandrakes could be used for sexual enticement.

COOKING/BAKING HACKS

325. Heat your pan before adding oil; then add the food. It will cook faster.

326. Sniff your spices before using. If you can't smell the aroma, it's probably gone stale and won't make anything spicy.

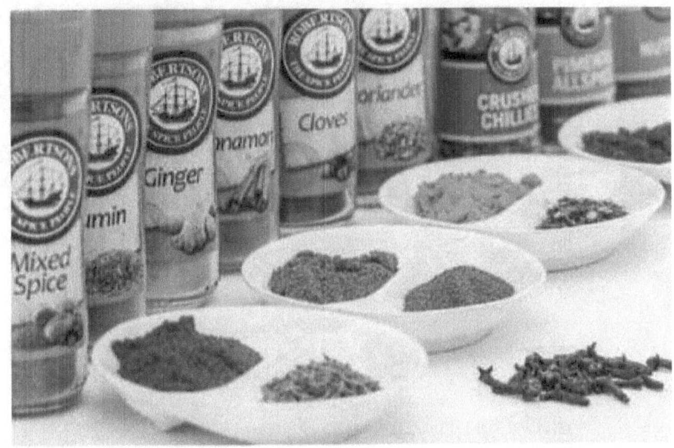

327. Test the freshness of your baking soda by putting a little in a bowl. Add vinegar. If it doesn't bubble up, it's too old.

328. Put a lid on the pot to make water boil faster.

329.   Freshen up stale chips, pretzels, or other salty snacks by warming in a low oven or microwaving 30-45 seconds. Let it stand for one minute to crisp up.

330.   Laying a wooden spoon across the top of your pan will keep the contents from boiling over.

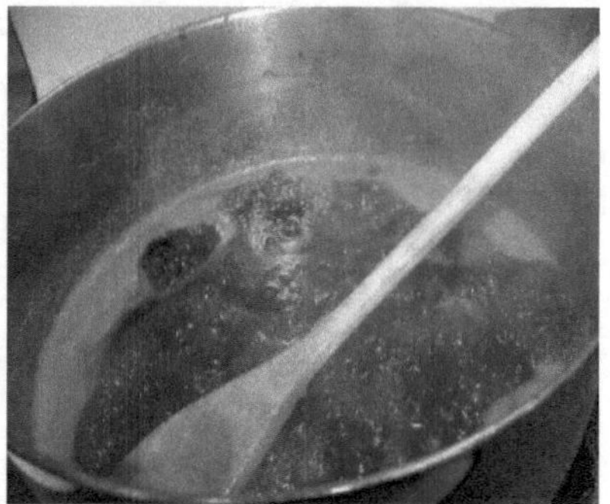

Picture by C.A. Simonson

331.   To keep your hands from smelling like garlic, rub your hands on stainless steel (like your sink) after handling garlic.

332.   Preheat your baking sheet along with the oven to roast veggies in half the time.

333.   Reheat pizza on top of the stove in a nonstick skillet on med-low heat. This keeps the crust crispy.

334. To warm up food more quickly in the microwave, arrange it in a circle on the plate. For spaghetti, make a "hole" in the center. For entrees such as lasagna, cut it into pieces.

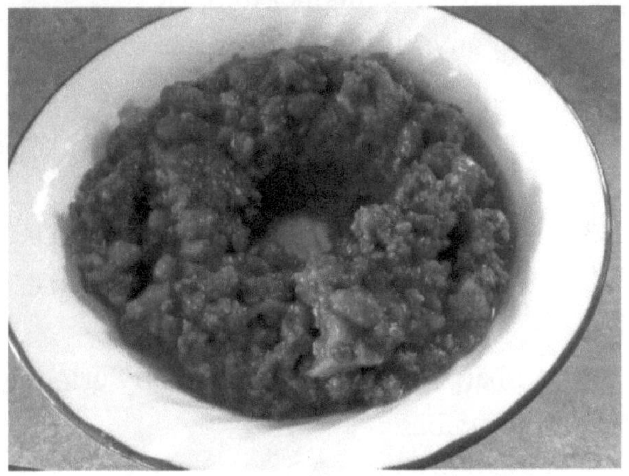

Picture by C.A. Simonson

335. Reheat pancakes, bread, or muffins in the microwave alongside a cup of water. The water keeps it from becoming tough or hard by adding moisture.

336. Use your waffle iron to make quick and easy hash browns.

337. Before measuring sticky substances like peanut butter, rinse the measuring cup with water first, or spray with oil.

338. Cut the pour spout off a used salt container to reuse on any Mason jar to create your own easy-pour container.

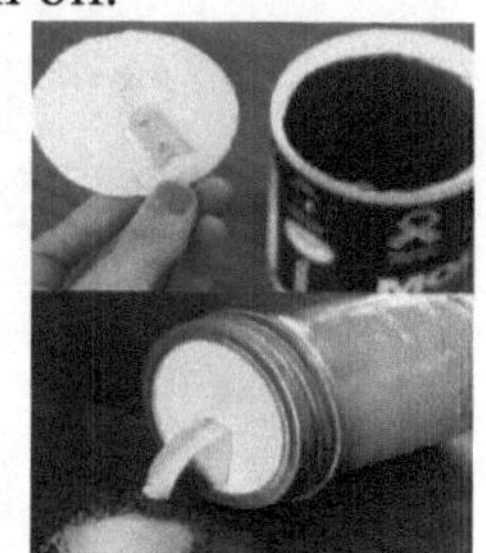

339. Transfer jelly or salad dressings to a squeeze bottle to prevent sticky jars.

340. Sharpen garbage disposals by grinding up ice cubes.

341. Grind your own spices with a coffee grinder.

342. Glasses stuck together? Put ice in the top glass, and then set both in hot water.

343. The easiest way to thaw frozen meat is still placing it in a sink or bowl full of cool water.

344. Burnt food in a pan? Let it cool, and then add hot water with vinegar and baking soda – or a capful of liquid fabric softener. Let it stand a few hours, and the burnt food will be easier to remove.

345. Pour salt on overflow of juices or pie filling in a hot oven for quick cleanup.

346. An empty small Pringles® can (half-can) works well to store cookies in a lunchbox.

347. Use less sugar by placing it in a shaker instead of a bowl.

348. Measure your milk for canned soup by using the can.

YOUR FOOD HACKS:

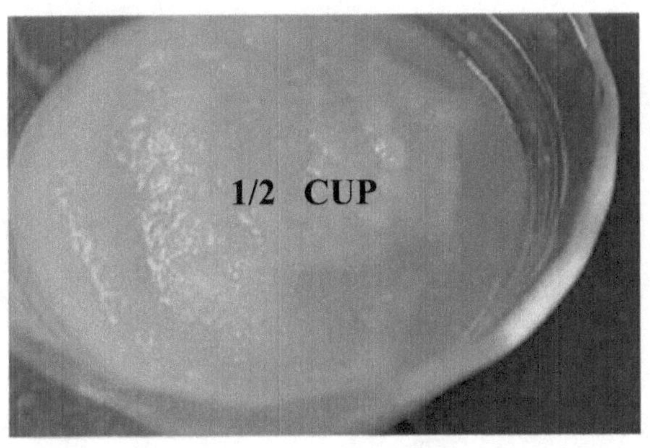

Substitutions

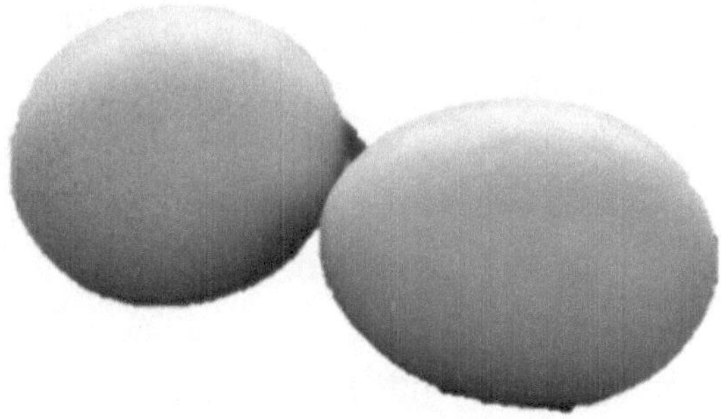

=

SUBSTITUTIONS

349. No buttermilk? Add a teaspoon of lemon juice to regular milk and wait for it to curdle. Works also for sour milk.

350. Greek yogurt can be a substitute for sour cream, heavy cream or mayonnaise. *(Fewer calories and better for you).

351. No baking powder? Use ¼ teaspoon of baking soda plus ½ teaspoon of cream of tartar for each teaspoon needed.

352. Substitute one square of chocolate with 3-4 Tablespoons of cocoa plus 1 Tablespoon of butter.

353. No brown sugar? Use 2 Tablespoons of molasses to ½ cup of granulated sugar for each ½ cup needed.

354. No tomato juice? Just add water to tomato sauce or ketchup.

355. No cornstarch? Tapioca or flour also works to thicken.

356. No barbeque sauce? Whip up your own with 1 cup ketchup and 1 cup of cola or grape jelly.

357. Make your own self-rising flour with 3 ½ cups regular flour, 1 ¾ tsp. baking powder, 1 ¾ tsp. baking soda, and 1 ¾ salt.

358. Mashed avocado replaces mayonnaise and is healthier for you!

359. No eggs? Use 1/4 c. of applesauce for each egg.

360. 1 mashed banana also equals 1 egg.

361. No sour milk for the recipe? Add ¾ tsp. baking soda into a cup of fresh milk. (Also works for buttermilk).

362. No vinegar? Use lemon or lime juice.

363. No whisk? Use a fork.

364. If you don't have a
cookie cutter for
round pastries, use
a glass.

365. No bread crumbs?
Use crushed saltine
crackers.

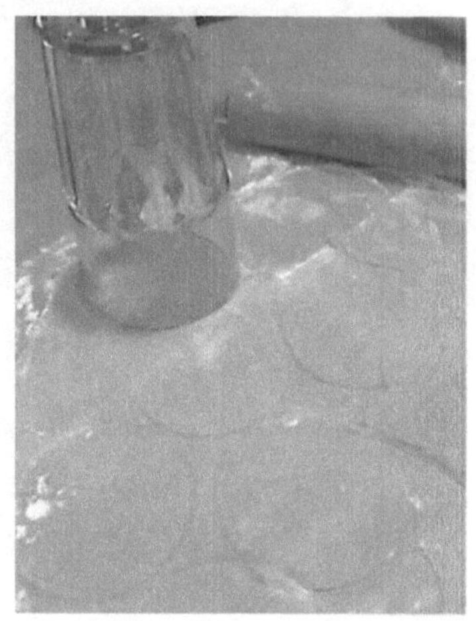

Picture by C.A. Simonson

Food:

A Beauty

Product

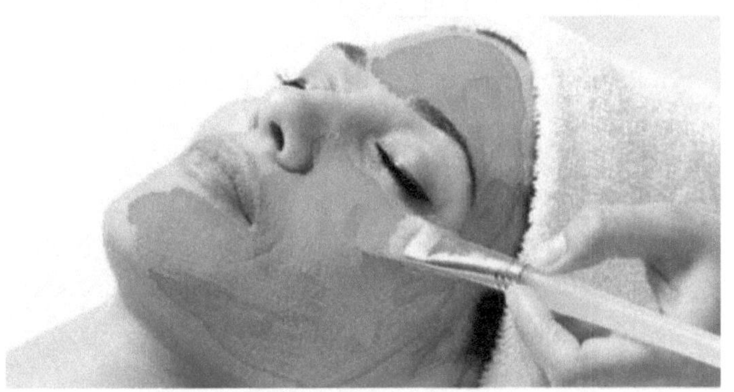

DID YOU KNOW?

Many of the ideas that follow were passed down from generation to generation. All-natural products often work the best for beauty inside and out

Ever remember your grandmother using sugar water or milk to stiffen a baby's hair?

In the 1960s, when I was a teen, many girls used to lather on Crisco, butter, or vegetable oil to get a beautiful brown tan. Problem was – many of them got 'fried' by the sun, too.

The ancient Egyptians used moldy bread to treat infections that arose from dirt in burn wounds.

Cleopatra used burnt almonds to draw on and shape her eyebrows and tinted her cheeks and lips with pomegranate juice.

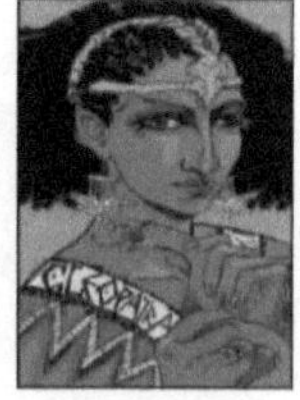

FOOD FOR BEAUTY

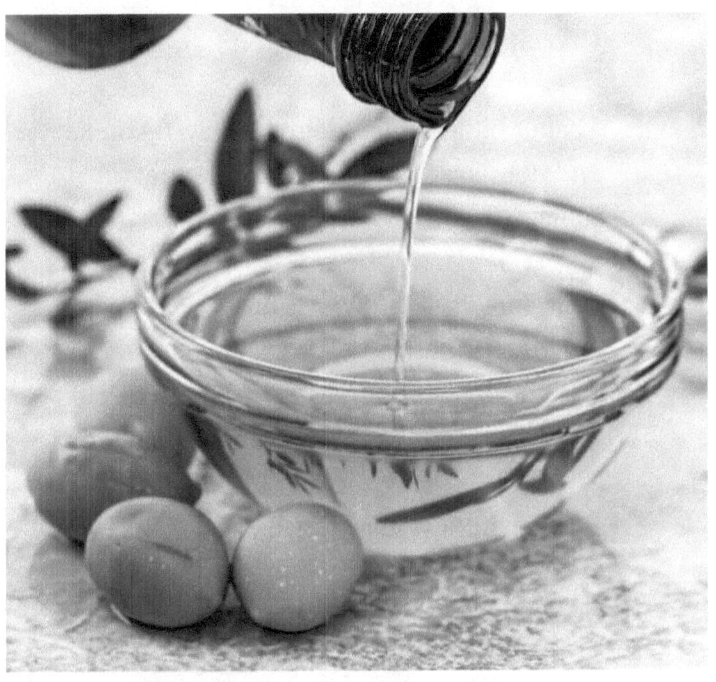

Ever wonder how bakers keep their hands supple after working in dough all day? Olive oil. It's a natural moisturizer. It has many other uses too.

SKIN SOFTENERS

1. Olive oil provides a closer shave than shaving cream.

2. Peanut butter makes a great shaving cream and nourishes your skin with natural moisturizers.

3. Exfoliate dry skin with a paste of ½ cup cooked oatmeal and ½ mashed banana. Before showering, massage the mixture on dry areas, and then wash away in the shower.

4. For the silkiest legs you'll ever have, use a sugar/oil scrub. Mix 2 ½ cups of sugar, 1 cup of olive or coconut oil, and 5 Tbsp. of lemon or lime juice. During your bath, soak for about five minutes and then shave your leg. Scrub with sugar/oil/juice mixture and then shave again. The second time removes dead skin. After your bath, dry and apply lotion for the silkiest legs ever.

5. Add a little olive oil to the bath water to leave skin soft and supple.

6. Say goodbye to cellulite by rubbing used coffee grounds over stubborn areas. Mix with oil to make a scrub and use in the shower. Rinse with soap and water.

7. Relieve aching muscles by adding 8 ounces of vinegar to a warm bath. Soak for 15 minutes.

8. Itchy skin from sunburn, bites, or poison ivy can be treated by soaking in a warm bath mixed with 1 cup of dry oatmeal and 8 ounces of vinegar for 15 minutes.

9. For an instant tonic on warm summer days, cool off with the peel of a cucumber.

FACIAL SCRUBS/CLEANSERS/ASTRINGENTS

10. Coconut oil is a natural wrinkle remover. It rebuilds skin tissue naturally. Apply as you would a face cream.

11. For DIY makeup remover, mix 3 Tablespoons of powdered milk with 1/3 cup of warm water in a jar and shake well. Add more water or powder as necessary to achieve the consistency of heavy cream. Apply to skin, and then wipe it off and rinse with water.

Mash up an over-ripe banana into a cream and apply it to your face for an all-natural face mask that moisturizes your skin and leaves it feeling fresh and soft. Let it set on your face for 20 minutes, and then rinse off with cool water.

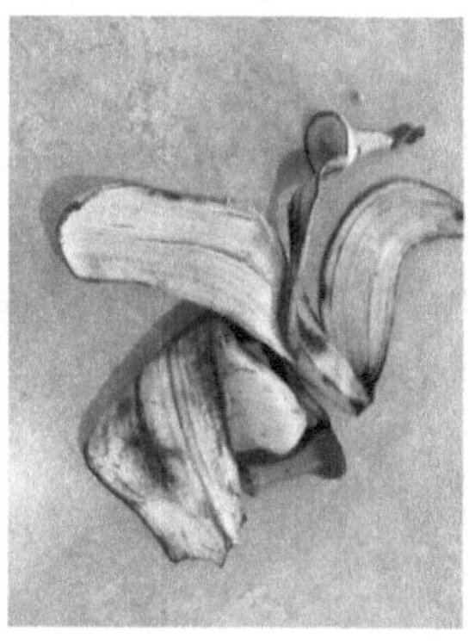

Picture by C.A. Simonson

12. Make your own astringent/skin toner by mixing 1 Tablespoon of apple cider vinegar with 2 cups of water. Use it as a rinse after a facial mask or washing to cleanse and tighten skin.

13. Get rid of blemishes overnight by applying a dab of honey. Place a Band-Aid® over it and watch it disappear.

14. For dry skin, make a facial mask from mashed avocado and olive oil. Massage into skin and leave it for 10 minutes. Rinse with warm water.

15. Use left-over rice water (after boiling rice) as a facial toner to shrink pores and lock in moisture.

16. Use brown sugar to make a facial scrub to remove dry skin and built-up bacteria in pores. 1 cup of brown sugar, ½ cup olive or coconut oil, ½ tsp. Vitamin E oil, and 1 tsp. vanilla extract. Massage on the face until the sugar melts. Rinse with warm water. This will keep for up to two months on the counter. This leaves the skin so soft and smooth – I tried it!

17. Banana peels will also heal bruises and cuts and eliminate rashes, itching, and even warts.

18. For relief from poison ivy, chicken pox, or
sunburn, pound four cups of Cheerios (or oatmeal) into a powder and add to a warm bath. Soak, relax, and feel relief.

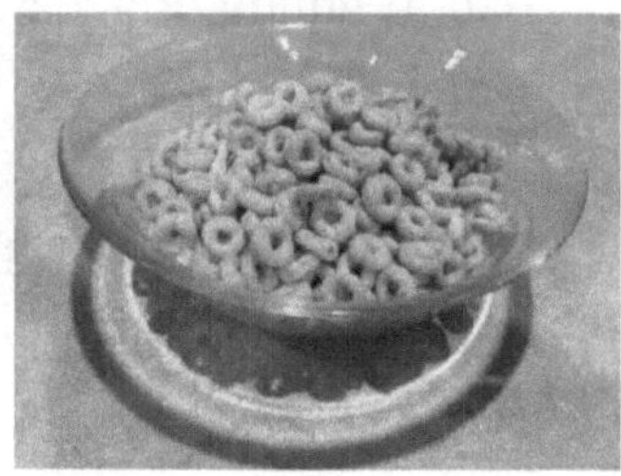

Picture by C.A. Simonson

19. Tighten pores and firm your facial skin with grapefruit and eggs. At bedtime, mash a peeled grapefruit and the whites of two eggs. Massage into face for 5 minutes, and then rinse.

20. Steam your face to open pores and deep-cleanse your skin. Pour boiling water into a bowl, place your face close to it with a towel over your head.

21. Mash 1 tomato and 1 avocado together and mix the pulp well. Spread the mixture on your face, and let it sit for 20 minutes. Rinse with warm water. For an even better cleanser, add oatmeal to the mixture.

22. Mayonnaise exfoliates and moistens skin. Massage it in after cleansing, let it rest for a few minutes, and then rinse.

23. Black tea makes a wonderful astringent. Splash on your face for a cool, refreshing feel.

24. To reduce pores on the skin, mix one tablespoon of tomato juice with two to four drops of fresh lime juice. Use a cotton ball 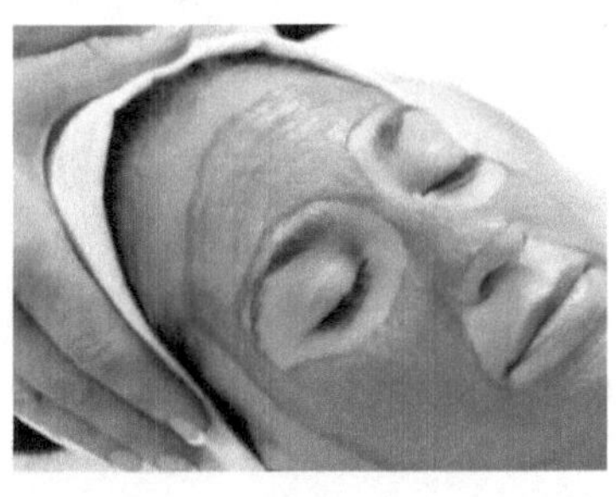 to apply to face using a circular motion. Leave on for 15 minutes, then rinse with cold water.

25. Treat dry, scaly skin with a paste of baking soda and olive oil. Apply to dry area and wait 3 minutes, then wash with warm water and soap.

26. Brown spots on your face/ Even them out with a lemon/sugar scrub. Grate lemon peel to get lemon zest. Let it dry and then grind to a powder. Mix in 1 tsp. sugar and add a little water. (The more water, the gentler the scrub). Massage into damp skin, rinse, and pat dry.

27. To treat pimples, make a paste of honey, flour, and vinegar. Dot the pimple and leave on overnight. Wash off in the morning.

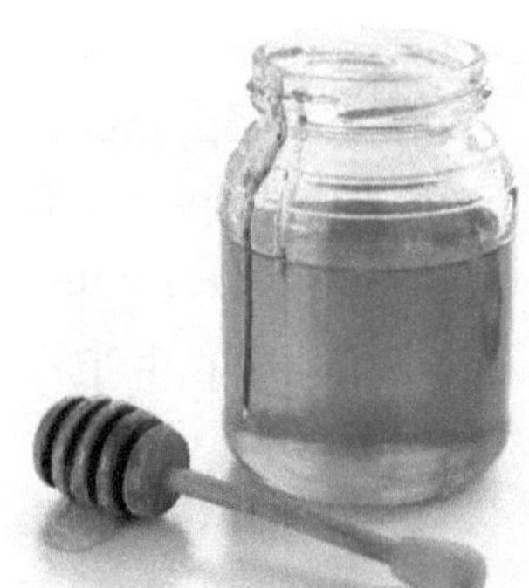

28. For acne, mix 1 tsp. vinegar with 10 tsp. water. Put into a well-sealed bottle. Dab on acne several times during the day. This shouldn't dry the skin.

29. A fix for oily skin, mix 1 tsp. salt into a spray bottle with warm water. Spritz face and blot dry.

30. For a fresh-feeling astringent, crush fresh
     mint leaves and pack them in a small jar.
     Cover with vinegar. Let stand two weeks and
     strain out the leaves. Use as a facial splash.

31. A cooling mask for too warm or rosy-red
     face is made of ½ cup applesauce and 1 Tbsp.
     honey. Apply, and then rinse.

32. Make a youthful mask that reduces fine lines
     and wrinkles with ½ banana, 2 Tbsp. honey
     and 2 Tbsp. heavy cream. Apply to face and
     rest for 10 minutes. Rinse with warm water.

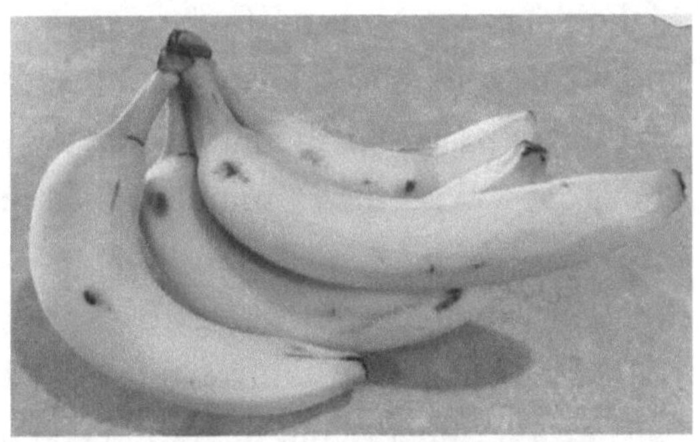

Picture by C.A. Simonson

33. Remove freckles or other dark spots by
     applying 3 parts of lemon juice to one part

olive oil. Pat onto troubled spots every day until they fade.

EYES

34.   Reduce baggy eye syndrome by placing chilled cucumber slices over eyes.

35.   Lighten the dark circles under your eyes with 1 tsp. turmeric, 1 tsp. tomato juice and ½ tsp. lime juice. Cream ingredients into a paste and dot under each eye. After five minutes, rinse.

36.   Make your own 'anti-puff' eye cream with ¼ cup whole milk and 4 Tbsp. baking soda. Mix into a paste, refrigerate. When cool, dab under eyes. Wait for 15 minutes, then rinse.

37.   Another way to de-puff baggy eyes is with cooled tea bags. Don't throw those used tea bags away! Squeeze out the liquid and then place the cooled bag over closed eyes 5-10 minutes.

38.   "Paint" orange juice around the eyes twice a day to reduce wrinkles, says an Old South remedy.

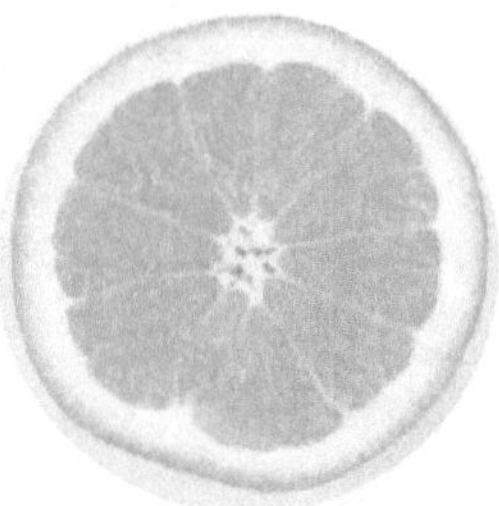

39.   Olive oil removes eye makeup easily and nourishes your skin.

40.   Use olive or coconut oil around the eyes at night to prevent fine lines and wrinkles, being especially careful not to get any in the eye or to stretch the skin around the eye.

HAIR

41.   Use a vinegar rinse when washing your hair to remove buildup from styling products, strengthen your hair, and leave it shiny and soft. It also balances the hair's pH levels.

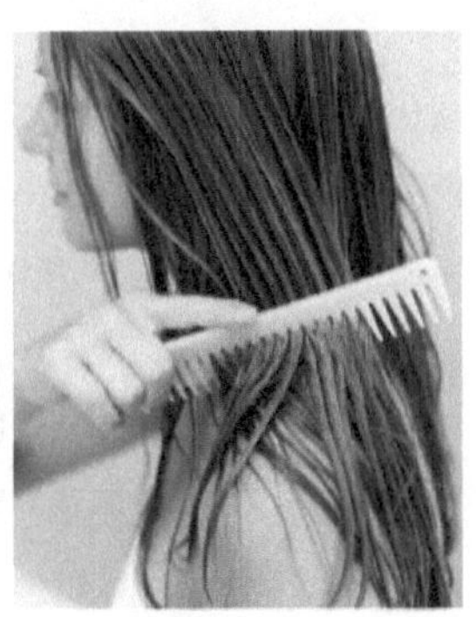

42. Combing a bit of olive oil through wet hair after a shower helps moisturize and defrizzes the dryness from winter harshness.

43. Use lemon juice as a highlighter for blond hair.

44. Add red highlights to your hair with ketchup! Pour into hair, work it in well, let it rest ten minutes, then rinse clean for natural red highlights.

45. For dandruff problems, briefly soak hair in a basin filled with water and ¼ cup vinegar before washing.

46. Ground-up oatmeal and baking soda make a quick dry shampoo when camping or there's no time to shower.

47. Vinegar rinse (1 Tbsp. vinegar to 1 gallon of water) helps minimize gray hair.

48. Remove gum from hair with peanut butter, mayonnaise, or whipped cream.

49.   For an itchy, flaky scalp, mash ½ banana, 2 Tablespoons of honey and a few drops of almond oil. Apply it to hair; let it set for 20 minutes under a shower cap (or plastic wrap); then rinse with water.

50.   Over-ripe bananas mashed into a cream will also make hair super soft because of all the natural oils and vitamins.

51.   My great-great aunt Ida claimed she kept her hair black without dye by drinking the water that all the vegetables were boiled in.

52.   Jell-O was often used as an Old South remedy for giving body to fine hair. Soften 1 Tbsp. unflavored gelatin in ¼ cup lemon juice. Add 1 cup of boiling water. When cool, comb through clean hair – your homemade mousse!'

53.   Pour strong, dark Indian tea over brown hair once a week, and your hair will not turn gray early.

54.   Hair frizzy from a permanent or sun can be tamed by rinsing with a vinegar solution (1 tsp. vinegar to 1 cup of warm water).

55.   For a fun, inexpensive, and *temporary* hair color, mix Kool-Aid® with your conditioner and apply to hair without rinsing. It will wash out the next time.

TEETH

56.   Apples are a natural toothbrush. Eat an apple after a meal!

57.   The inside peel of a banana will whiten your teeth. Gently rub the inside on your teeth for about two minutes. It's the vitamins in the banana peel that make the difference.

58.   Club soda works as a denture cleanser.

59.   Brighten dentures by soaking in straight vinegar.

60.   A mixture of salt and baking soda makes 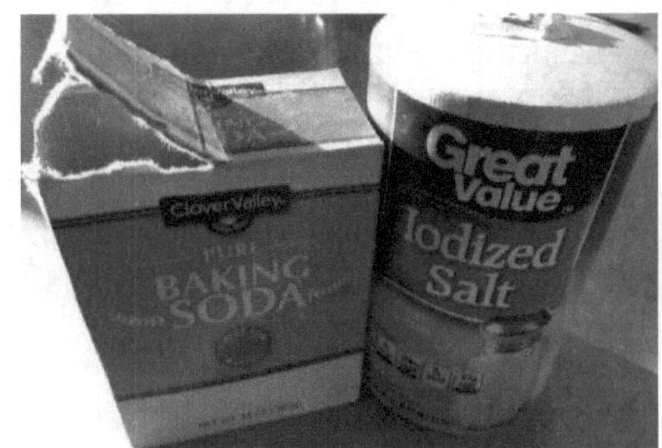

an excellent toothpaste that whitens teeth and removes plaque. (Crush salt into sand-like texture first). Keep in an air-tight container.

61.   Make your own minty toothpaste with 1 Tbsp. baking soda, 1 Tbsp. salt, 1 tsp. lemon juice and 1 drop of peppermint or spearmint oil. White teeth and fresh minty breath!

62.   Remove oil, tar, or grease from hands with Mayonnaise.

NAILS, HANDS & FEET

63.   Keep nails supple by soaking them in a bowl of 2 Tbsp. crushed pineapple mixed with 1 egg yolk for 5 minutes, then wash with warm water.

64.   Keep feet odors at bay by sprinkling a little baking soda in your shoes.

65.   Yellowed fingernails? Rub a wedge of lemon over fingernails to whiten them, or soak in a bowl of lemon juice.

66.   Soaking your feet in a solution of black tea will make foot odor disappear.

67.   Remove corns and calluses by covering the rough areas with cotton balls soaked in vinegar. Secure with a band-aid or tape and leave on overnight. Repeat until problem areas disappear.

68.   Dry, cracked heels? Make your own foot cream with dry rice (grind or blend into a powder), raw honey, olive oil, and enough apple cider vinegar to make a

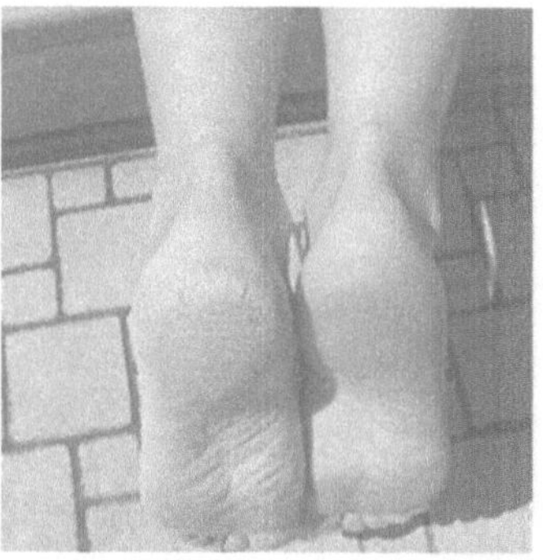

thick paste. After soaking feet for 20 minutes, gently massage with this paste, and then rinse.

69. Soaking your feet in a solution of warm water and mustard will soothe aching, tired feet.

70. To keep athlete's foot at bay, add 4 ounces of oregano leaves into water (1/2 to 3/4 bucket) to cover your feet. Soak your feet in this solution at least 2 times daily. Prepare it fresh each time in order to keep it fungus free.

71. Dusting the feet with cornstarch will keep feet dry, help prevent foot odor, and athlete's foot.

72. Coconut oil has anti-fungal properties. Use it on infected areas of the skin to help heal.

YOUR BEAUTY TRICKS:

Food: A Cleaner

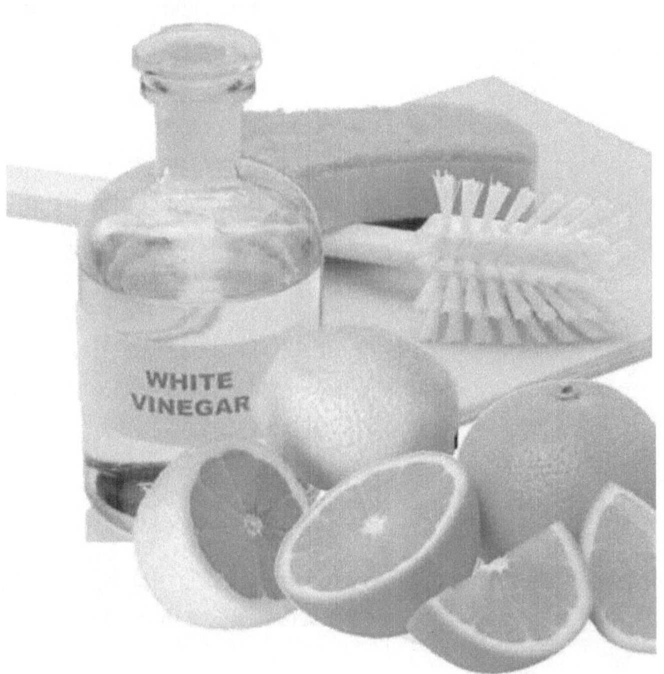

DID YOU KNOW?

Clean with white vinegar: use apple cider vinegar for beauty.

✠

Crisco shortening is actually 80% liquid oil. It was invented in 1911 by a candlemaker (Proctor) and a soap maker (Gamble).

✠

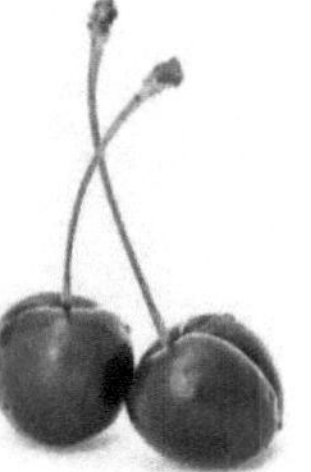

According to sciencelive.com, carminic acid is a common red food dye that can be found in Skittles, maraschino cherries, raspberry and strawberry-flavored junk food. Carminic acid also happens to be made from the crushed carcasses of a South American beetle.

✠

Gummy candies get that glossy sheen with a coating of carnauba wax, the same stuff used on cars to make them shiny.

✠

Wasabi is a very expensive Japanese condiment. Most of the wasabi served in restaurants in the US is simply green-dyed horseradish.

FOOD AS A CLEANER

All you really need is lots of vinegar, lemons, and baking soda!

HAND CLEANER

73. Use sugar, along with soap and water, as a buffer to wash your hands when stained from gardening.

74. Lemon juice removes odors from hands.

CLOTHES

75. To keep bright colored clothes from fading, soak them overnight in strong salt water.

76. Sour milk will whiten shoe laces. Let them soak overnight, and then wash.

77. Remove ink stains on clothing by soaking overnight in milk.

78.　Make your towels fluffy and absorbent again by washing them with hot water and one cup of vinegar. Then wash again with hot water and one-half cup of baking soda.

79.　Remove dried blood from clothing by soaking in Coke, and then wash as usual.

80.　Empty a can of Coke in the washer with a load of greasy clothes along with detergent to remove grease easily.

Picture by C.A. Simonson

81.　Make your own environmentally-safe bleach by mixing equal amounts of lemon juice and baking soda.

82.　Mix equal amounts of lemon juice and baking soda to get rid of underarm stains.

83.　Remove grass stains from clothes by soaking in vinegar ½ hour before washing.

84. If you use a box of baking soda in your refrigerator as a deodorizer, change it out every 4-6 months. But don't throw it away! Toss ½ cup with your laundry detergent for cleaner clothes! It makes your detergent work better.

85. Keep clothes from fading by adding a teaspoon of pepper to the wash.

86. A cup of lemon juice added to the wash cycle will whiten clothes.

87. Club soda is great for removing stains from fabric. Apply with a cloth, blot, and voila! Stain is gone.

88. Cigarette smells can be removed from clothes by soaking in a solution of 4 Tbsp. baking soda and 1 quart of water before washing.

89. Brighten colors and prevent colors from running in the wash cycle by adding 3-4 tsp. of salt to the wash.

SHOES

90. Give your shoes a professional-looking shine by rubbing the shoe with the inside of a banana peel. Buff with a soft cloth afterward.

91. Clean patent leather by dabbing on milk. Let it dry, then buff it off.

92. Clean suede shoes with baking soda applied with a soft brush. Let it sit a while, and then brush off.

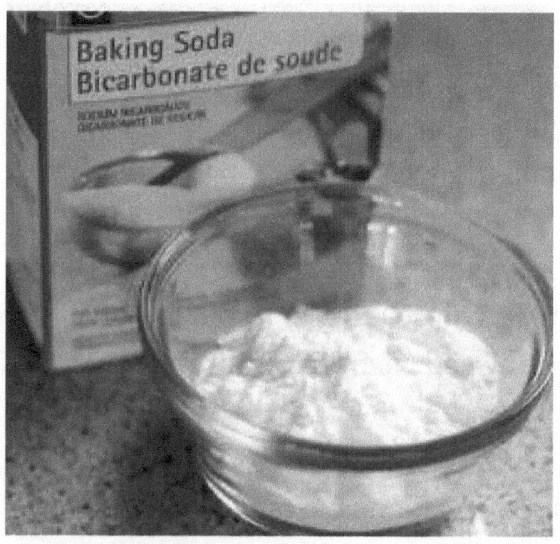

93. Clean rubber-soled tennis shoes with baking soda on a wet sponge.

94. Remove scuff marks on shoes with a paste made of baking soda and water.

95. Rubbing cucumber on your shoes gives a quick polish, but also makes them water resistant.

ALL AROUND HOME

96. Make your own "green" cleaner by soaking orange or lemon peels in a quart jar of white vinegar. Let it sit for two weeks, throw the orange peels away and pour the vinegar into a spray bottle.

97. Remove crayon marks from walls with a damp sponge dipped in baking soda.

98. Remove stains from laminated countertops with a paste of baking soda and water. Apply, let dry, then rub off and rinse.

99. Clean greasy fingerprints off walls with bread.

100. Brighten faded carpets or rug by rubbing a cloth soaked with a strong salt solution over them.

101. Pour sour milk down the toilet to help clean the septic tank.

102. Sprinkle your carpet with salt if you suspect fleas have invaded from your pets. Let stand a few hours and then vacuum. Repeat weekly for six weeks.

103. Put salt in your vacuum cleaner bag to kill off any flea eggs which may have been vacuumed up.

104. Soap scum is loosened quickly on shower doors with white vinegar. Spray on and let dry. Respray to dampen, and then wipe down for a shine.

105. De-clog drains the environmentally-safe way by pouring a can of cola down the drain. Let it sit for about one hour, and then run hot water through the drains.

106.   Clean and whiten grout with lemon and white vinegar. To 7 cups of water, add ½ c. baking soda, 1/3 c. lemon juice, and ¼ c. vinegar. Put it into a spray bottle, spray the grout and allow to sit a minute or two, and then scrub.

107.   Cucumber removes the crayon and marker prints on walls.

108.   Remove hard water and mineral deposit around sink and tub faucets by covering them with a paper towel soaked in vinegar. Let sit for an hour, then wipe down with a damp sponge.

109.   Moldy or mildewed areas of the bathroom such as shower curtains can be removed with vinegar. Spray on. Let sit a few minutes, and then wipe down.

110.   Forget the harsh chemicals to clean the tub. Simply pour salt on a half of grapefruit and scrub that tub clean!

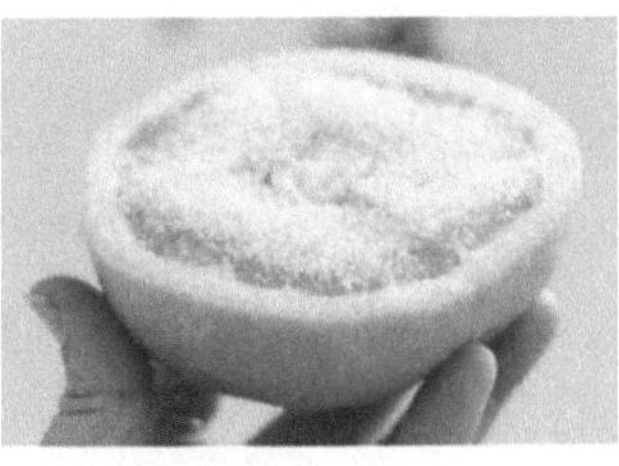

111. Clean your windows with white vinegar for a non-streak shine. Put into a spritz bottle for easy application.

112. My Aunt Ruby said adding a little cornstarch to the water when washing windows makes streak-free glass. (A gallon of warm water to ½ cup cornstarch). Polish with a dry cloth.

113. Tea will shine a wooden floor.

FURNITURE

114. Olive oil can be used as a polish for silverware or stainless steel.

115. As a wood furniture cleaner, mix two parts olive oil with one part lemon juice or vinegar. Gently rub furniture, and then buff off.

116. Make scuffs and scratches disappear on wooden furniture by rubbing a piece of walnut into it.

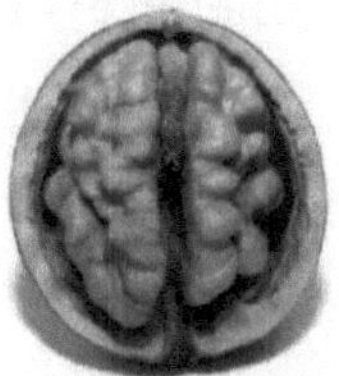

117.   Remove an ink stain from leather furniture by
        rubbing on a bit of baking soda. Leave on
        until the ink is absorbed and then brush off.

118.   A fresh grease stain on cloth furniture can be
        removed with equal parts of baking soda and
        salt. Rub lightly, leave it for a few hours, and
        then vacuum.

119.   Clean vinyl upholstery with a paste of baking
        soda and water. Rub it on, allow to dry, and
        then wipe it off.

120.   Baking soda deodorizes carpets. Sprinkle in,
        let sit overnight, and then vacuum.

121.   Coffee, chocolate, or cola stains on the carpet
        can be cleaned with 1-part white vinegar to
        2-parts water. Sponge on and blot until the
        stain is gone.

122.   Store baking soda in old pantyhose 'sachets'
        in closets or luggage to prevent musty odors.

123. White vinegar kills mildew. Mix equal parts
      of vinegar and water and use where you
      suspect mildew. Let it dry into the area.

124. Sprinkle salt on a red wine spill on a carpet.
      Let it sit for 15 minutes and then clean with
      1-part white vinegar and 2 parts water.

125. Remove a scald or water mark from wooden
      furniture with a paste of vegetable shortening
      and a pinch of salt. Apply to mark with a soft
      cloth and then buff lightly as it's wiped off.

126. Reduce garbage can odors by sprinkling the
      bottom with baking soda each time the
      garbage bag is replaced.

127. No dusting spray? Boil a few cups of water,
      then steep 2 tea bags until it cools. Pour into
      a spray bottle with a teaspoon of lemon juice.

128. Make your own carpet freshener with 1 cup
      of herbs (like lavender or rosemary), 1 tsp.
      cinnamon, 1 tsp. clove, and 1 tsp. baking
      soda. Combine and sprinkle over the carpet.
      Let it sit for a few minutes, and then vacuum.

129. Mayonnaise will remove white rings on furniture. Rub in, allow to sit for a few minutes, then wipe off, & buff.

DISHES/POTS & PANS

130. Soak a sponge in a shallow dish of vinegar to keep it from going sour in humid weather.

131. Clean darkened aluminum pans by boiling them ten minutes in a mixture of two teaspoons of cream of tartar mixed in one quart of water.

132. Darkened pots from boiling water can be cleaned with tomato juice or spaghetti sauce by boiling in the same pot.

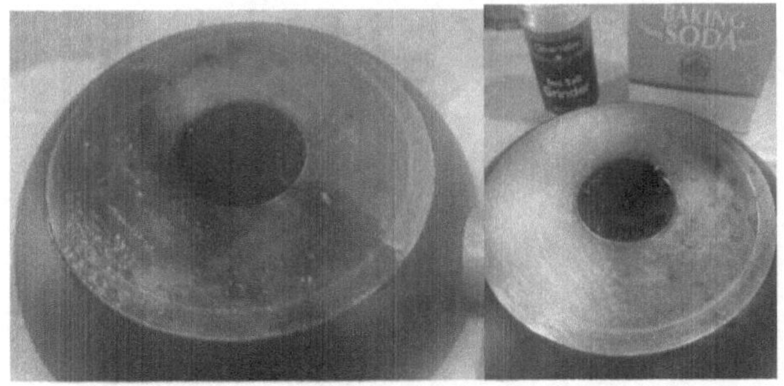

Picture by C.A. Simonson

133.   Rub ketchup on the bottom of a darkened stainless steel pan; add a little baking soda and some salt. Let sit for a few minutes, and then scrub off for a beautiful shine.

134.   Get rid of cracks in fine China dishes by covering them with boiling milk. Allow to sit until milk is cooled. Cracks all disappear.

135.   Peanut butter removes sticky labels.

136.   Club soda removes stains from coffee mugs and silver.

137.   Brighten aluminum pans with cream of tartar.

138.   Add one Tablespoon of lemon juice to your dishwasher rinse for spot-free glasses.

139.   Polish brass and stainless steel with a lemon juice and salt mixture.

140.   Remove the oily orange stains from plasticware by cleaning with a paste of baking soda. Let it sit for a few hours, then wash with soap and water.

141.   Clean copper-bottomed pans with ketchup.

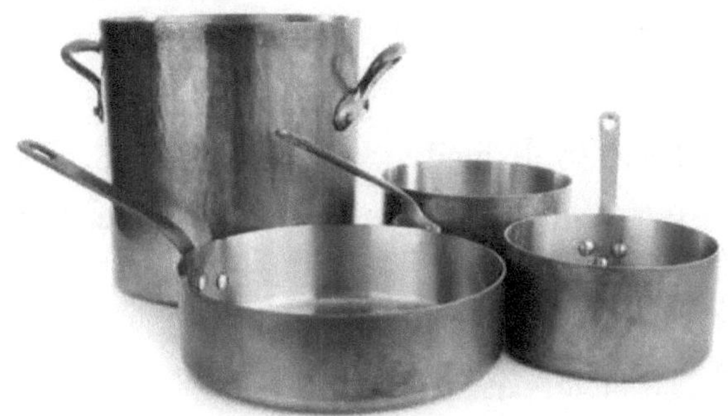

142.   Polish copper-bottomed pans with lemon juice.

143.   Clean burned-on messes from a broiler by adding 2 cups vinegar to ¼ cup sugar to the burned pan while it is warm. Soak for an hour, and then clean as usual.

144.   Make your sterling silver sparkle again by soaking in lemon-lime soda.

145.   Egg shells can be used as a make-shift steel wool to help clean pans – a trick particularly useful while camping.

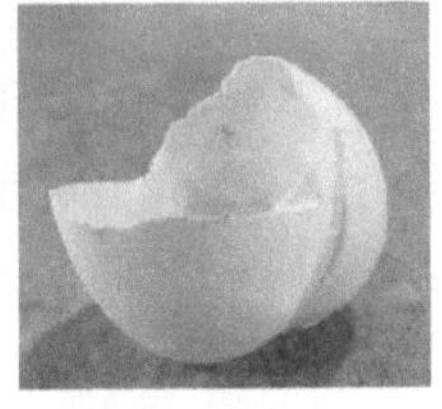

Picture by C.A. Simonson

146.   Clean the residue or water stains from the inside of a slim vase with vinegar and baking soda.

147.   Never polish silver again. Just soak overnight in sour milk and wash clean the next day.

148.   To clean cast-iron pans, add 2 tablespoons of oil and place on medium heat. Once the pan is heated, pour in 3 Tablespoons of salt. Use a tong to hold a 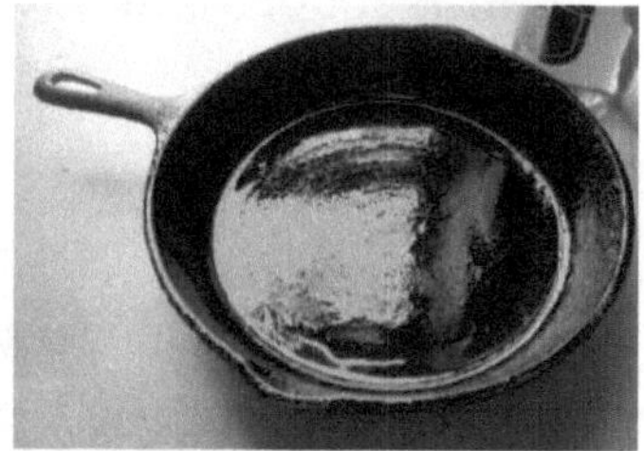 paper towel and scour until clean. Then, rinse and coat with vegetable oil to cure.

APPLIANCES

149.   Wipe bath and kitchen fixtures with club soda to make them shine.

150.   Clean the rubber seals of your refrigerator/freezer with undiluted

vinegar. This prevents mildew and reduces any odor. Use a toothbrush to get into the folds.

151.   Place a small bowl of vinegar on the top rack of a dishwasher while washing to avoid spots and streaks on glasses.

152.   Put a bowl of lemon juice and water into the microwave and heat. The steam will loosen stains and grime, making it much easier to clean.

153.   Erase hard water stains on stainless steel by rubbing with a lemon wedge.

154.   Clean your coffee grinder by grinding up uncooked rice.

155.   Clean residue from an iron by ironing (with no steam) over plain paper sprinkled with salt.

156.   Cucumbers are great for cleaning
        stainless steel, removing tarnish and
        bringing back shine.

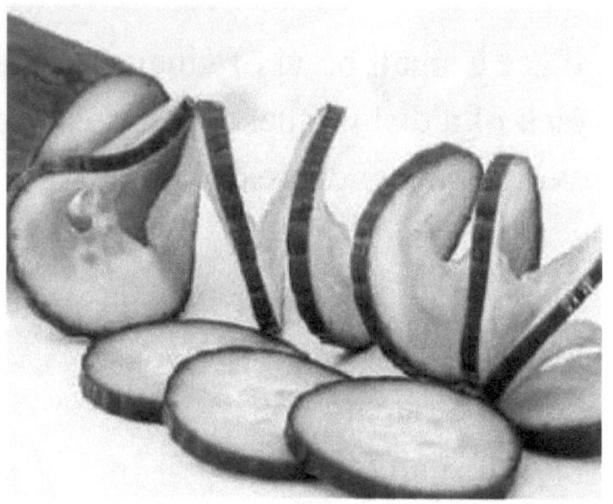

157.   Hard water spots and stains can be
        removed from the inside of a dishwasher
        with lemonade mix. Pour the dry powder
        into the detergent cup and run the
        dishwasher while empty.

158.   Get rid of burnt popcorn smell from the
        microwave. Heat a small glass dish or
        vinegar for 5 minutes. Remove and wipe
        down the inside.

159.   Deodorize and clean the inside of your
        microwave from splatters by boiling a

small bowl of vinegar for 3 minutes. Remove the dish and wipe out.

160. Clean the inside of your clothes washer by running a hot water cycle with 1 quart of vinegar.

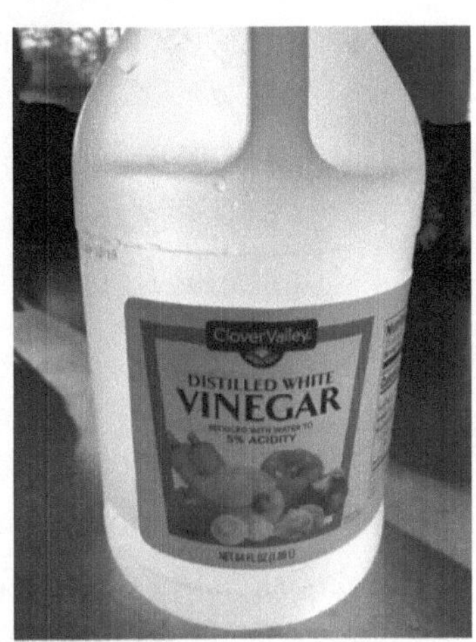

161. One-half cup of vinegar added to towels during the wash cycle makes them softer and brighter.

162. Clean your blender with ice. Fill half-full of soapy water and a handful of crushed ice, then run on high.

163. Go eco-friendly by using white vinegar instead of a rinse aide in your dishwasher.

164. Clean the buildup inside your coffeemaker by brewing a cycle of cold

water with ¼ cup white vinegar. Repeat 2-3 times, then run through fresh cold water to get rid of the vinegar smell.

165.   When ingredients spill over in the oven or on the stovetop, pour salt on the spill. It will stop it from burning and avoid smoke.

166.   Clean and deodorize your garbage disposal by pouring one-half cupful of baking soda down the drain followed by one cup of white vinegar. When foaming subsides, run hot water down the drain.

Weird Uses for Food

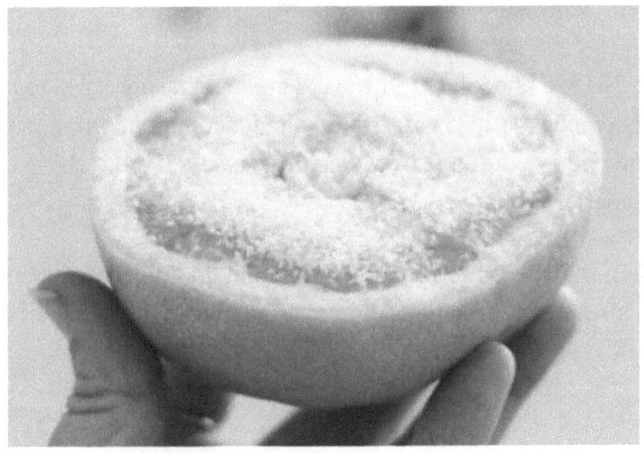

You Won't Believe

DID YOU KNOW?

The "stuff" that forms on vinegar is called 'mother.' It is cellulose, a natural by-product of harmless vinegar bacteria. It will not form on pasteurized bottles.

✠

Coca-Cola was invented in 1885 – as a cure for headaches. Called French Wine Cola, the temperance movement of the 1880s forced the inventor to remove the wine from the coca syrup. When the liquid was diluted with soda water, "soda pop" was created! Where I grew up, we called it pop, not soda pop.

✠

In 2015, a chocolatier in Ireland created "raspberry blood chocolate" with 2% pig's blood and a combination of raspberry and cherry cordial filling. Needless to say, it didn't hit the markets.

Sodium caseinate, an ingredient in the non-dairy whipped cream, is also the ingredient used in making glue. This whipped cream will keep for weeks in the refrigerator.

✠

Spam (the spicy canned ham) served as rations for troops during WWII and fueled the Normandy invasion. Margaret Thatcher called it the "wartime delicacy."

WEIRD USES FOR FOOD YOU WON'T BELIEVE

INSIDE THE HOUSE

167. Eggs are awful to clean up when dropped. Easy way? Sprinkle salt over it; wait for it to dry and then use a dustpan to sweep it up.

168. Rub a cucumber slice over your mirror to prevent it from fogging up during a shower.

169. Use a piece of bread to pick up broken glass.

170. Half of a potato will help remove a broken light bulb from its socket.

171. Fill small holes in walls with a paste of flour and water.

172. Clean hairbrushes and combs easily by soaking them in hot water combined with vinegar and baking soda for a few hours.

173. Stop the smoke alarm! Dampen a dishtowel in vinegar and wave in the smoky area.

174. Setting a bowl of vinegar in a room that's being freshly painted removes the paint odor.

175. Sharpen a knife more quickly by dipping it in vinegar before applying it to the whetstone.

176. Clean bricks on a fireplace with straight vinegar and a wire brush.

177. When painting a room, set a raw onion in the middle of the room to absorb the odors.

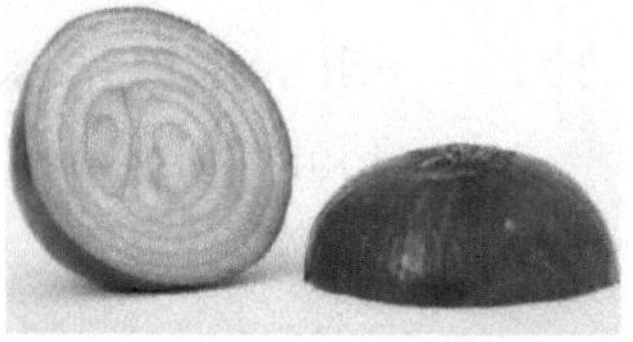

178. My grandmother claimed setting a raw onion in a room would also absorb bacteria, thus preventing sickness.

179. Keep cockroaches at bay by combining a mixture of powdered sugar and baking soda. Place in corners and dark places in soda bottle caps. The sugar draws them, the baking soda makes them explode.

180. Mix flour and water together for paste. It was how my mother put up wallpaper, and how I pasted in my scrapbook as a child.

181. Use a little bit of sugar on a burnt tongue to ease pain.

"Just a spoon full of sugar..."

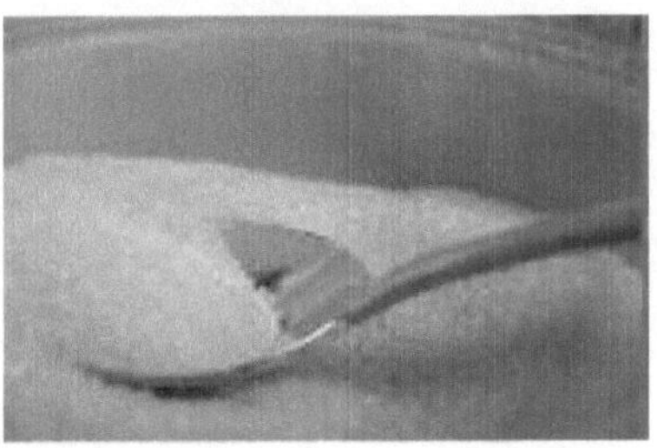

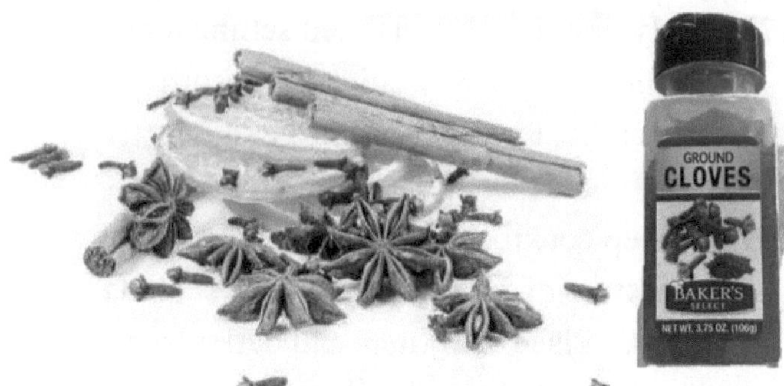

182.   A pinch of powdered cloves will ease the
        pain of a toothache.

183.   Spearmint or peppermint will help an
        upset stomach or nausea.

184.   Coconut oil works wonders on a diaper
        rash.

185.   Remove a stuck-on ring by lathering the
        finger with Mayonnaise or peanut butter.

OUTSIDE THE HOUSE

186. Mix equal parts of baking soda and yellow cornmeal to clean up light oil spills in your garage. Let dry, and then sweep away.

187. Use mayonnaise to remove sticky bumper stickers. Spread it liberally on the bumper sticker; wait for thirty minutes, and then rub off with a clean towel.

188. Soak a cotton ball in vanilla or cinnamon oil. Put it into a salt shaker and store in your car for an easy air freshener.

189. Bring a hardened paint brush back to life by soaking in ½ gallon water mixed with 1 cup baking soda and ¼ cup white vinegar.

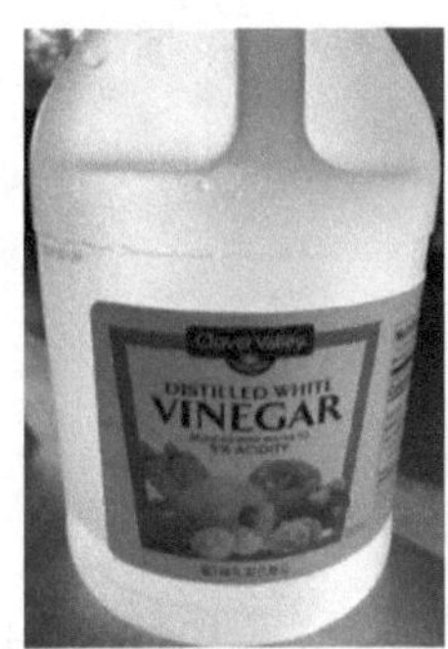

190. Remove rust from tools by soaking overnight in vinegar.

191. Remove rust from bicycle handlebars or tire rims with a paste of 6 Tbsp. salt mixed with 2 Tbsp. lemon juice. Rub into the rusty areas with a dry cloth. Rinse, and then dry.

192. A paste of vinegar and cornstarch will take the sting out of a bee or wasp sting or bug bite.

193. Ketchup is great for making skunk odor disappear, but what if you run out?

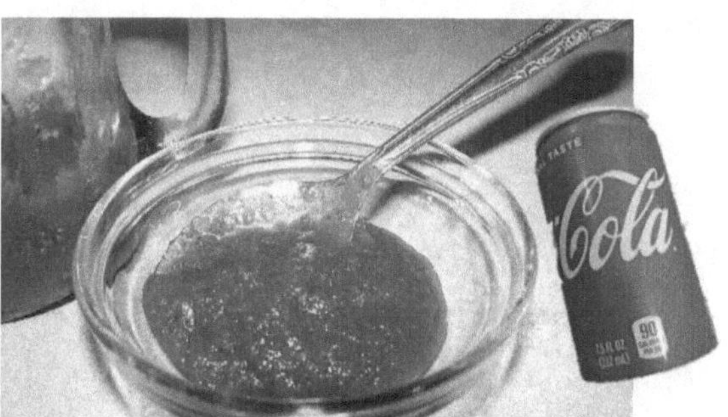

Picture by C.A. Simonson

Use a can of cola.
Rub it in, let it sit for 30 minutes, and then wash it out. (Be cautious to only use it on dark-furry animals).

194.   Soothe the rash of poison ivy with a vinegar compress. One-half cup of vinegar to 1 pint of water, chilled, will help.

195.   Spritz lemon juice on your skin or clothes as an insect repellent.

196.   Crumble eggshells and put them in your compost or in your garden for perfectly fertilized soils which naturally repel slugs.

197.   Geraniums, begonias, hydrangeas like alkaline soil. Water them occasionally with a solution of 3 Tbsp. of baking soda to 1 quart of water.

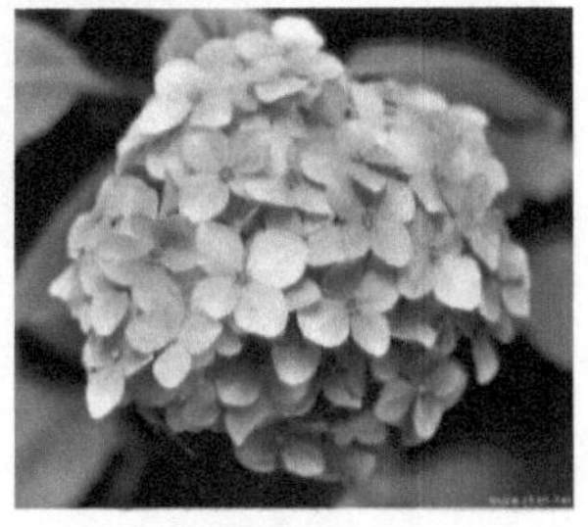

198.   Spray a light coat of vegetable oil on tropical flowers to keep them fresh longer.

199. Baking soda sprinkled around tomato plants will sweeten them.

200. A half of an egg shell makes a good starter for new plants. Put a little dirt in the egg shell, plant the seed, and stick back in the carton. Set the carton in the sunshine and watch them grow.

201. Kill weeds between the cracks in your sidewalk or driveway by a mixture of 1quart boiling water with 2 Tbsp. salt and 5 Tbsp. vinegar. Pour it on weeds while hot.

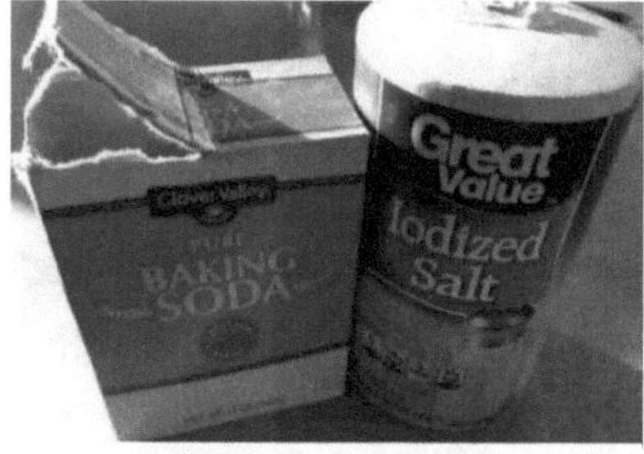

Picture by C.A. Simonson

202. Pancake syrup will revive an ailing plant (2 Tablespoons to the soil once a month).

203. Syrup also keeps your real Christmas tree fresh longer (add it to the water daily).

204. Shine plant leaves with Mayonnaise.

205. Tea is also a good fertilizer for roses.

206. A strong salt solution mixed with soapy water will kill poison ivy.

207. Tea leaves are a natural means to keep mosquitoes away. Dampen leaves to the areas you want to keep insect-free with tea.

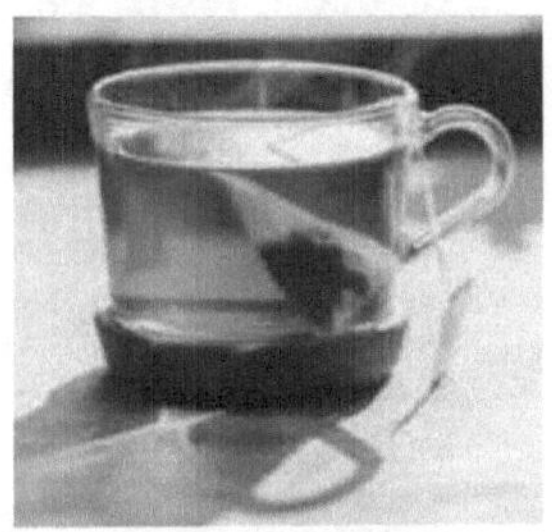

If you liked this book, I'd love to hear about it. Write a review on Amazon.com. Scroll to the bottom of the page where you bought the book and jot your thoughts.

OTHER BOOKS BY C.A. SIMONSON

Read the Journey Home trilogy, Christian romance/adventure/mystery/drama – all rolled into one. Seven children abandoned by their drunken father have to separate to survive. What will they do? Where will they go? Will they ever find each other again?

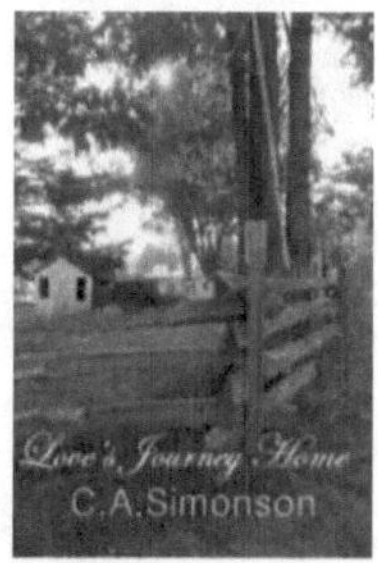 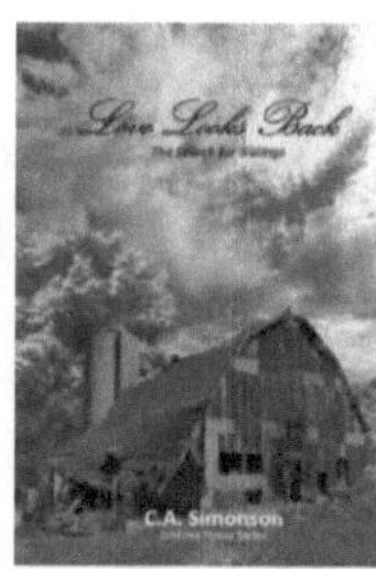 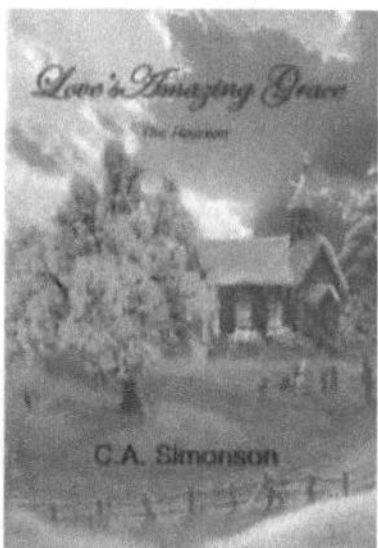

Available in print, e-book, and audio at Amazon.

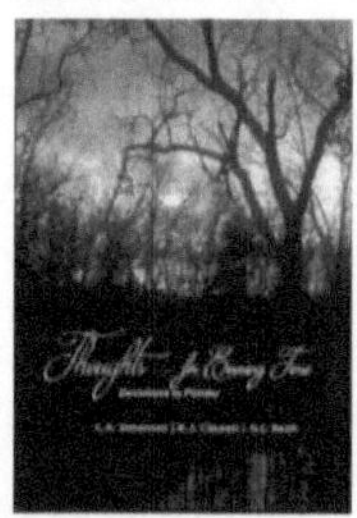 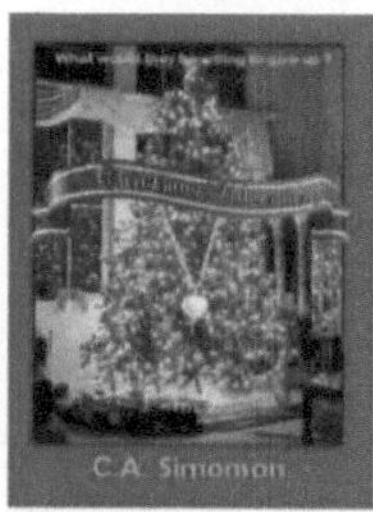 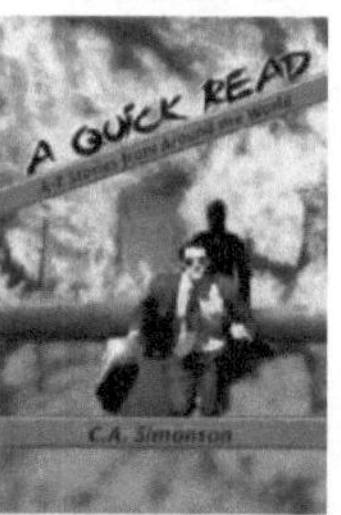

Thoughts for Evening Time- a 5-minute devotional
The Christmas Adventure –a novella
A Quick Read -54 short stories written from A-Z

ABOUT THE AUTHOR

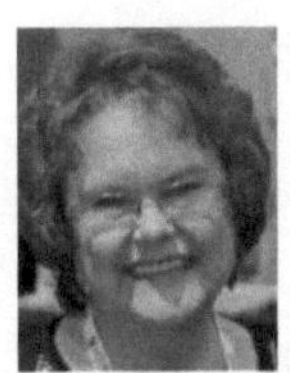 I have been collecting and gathering thoughts, hints, and tips for over twenty years from every place I've lived. Living in four different states brought new ideas and tips. My theory has always been – if it can be achieved quicker, easier, and simpler and still get the same great results or better, why not do it? I am a cook who likes to use every tidbit and not waste anything, because there *must* be a use for it *somewhere*. Many of these I've tried and proved; some are still waiting to be explored.

I hope you have gleaned some new ideas and helps. Maybe you have more of your own you'd like to share. Contact me at casimonson@hotmail.com and let me know! Check out my food website at

www.kitchentipsandtreasures.wordpress.com

for tips, hints, recipes, stories, and more.

✠

C.A. Simonson lives in southwest Missouri in the beautiful Ozarks. When she is not writing another book or helping other authors succeed, she is fishing in their backyard pond or making a quilt.